A Practitioner's Guide To
ERECTILE DYSFUNCTION
A Contemporary Clinical Approach

Dr. (Prof.) Rajan Bhonsle, M.D.
Senior Consultant in Sexual Medicine and Counsellor
Hon. Professor & Head of the Department of Sexual Medicine
KEM Hospital & Seth G.S. Medical College, Mumbai
Diplomate, American Board of Sexology &
American College of Sexologists

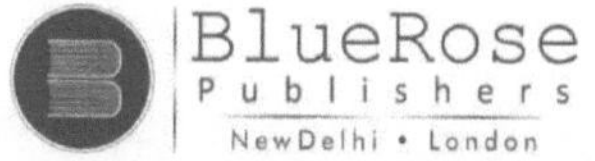

First Published in February 2022

ISBN: 978-93-93899-11-8

BLUEROSE PUBLISHERS

www.bluerosepublishers.com

info@bluerosepublishers.com

+91 8882 898 898

Cover Design:

Aveek

Typographic Design:

Tanya Raj Upadhyay

Distributed by: BlueRose, Amazon, Flipkart

PREFACE

Erectile Dysfunction (ED) is one of the most prevalent and complex problems that we see in the field of sexual medicine. Practically every man irrespective of his age, race, nationality, health or financial status experiences it sometime or the other in his life. Starting from adolescent boys to men in their 60s, 70s and 80s, I have seen the entire spectrum of men struggling with this problem with the widest possible range of causes (etiology), from psychogenic to organic to iatrogenic. Each of these cases needs an individual and specific analysis, diagnosis and treatment. I haven't found a single book that encompasses all aspects, approaches and options concerning the diagnosis and management of ED. All the information concerning ED is scattered and randomly spread across the sexology literature. I have put it all together in a systematic and *easy-to-unfold* manner in this book, to guide every qualified medical practitioner practicing with integrity, irrespective of his specialization or experience.

One of the serious issues that we face in India is 'quackery', particularly in the field of sexual medicine. There are a large number of unqualified quacks who pose themselves as sexologists. They not just exploit patients, but also indulge in potentially harmful practices. Just by becoming a member of a certain association, many of them start calling themselves as sexologists. A significant number of them do not even have a primary MBBS degree. This is a matter of concern.

One of the reasons to write this book is to eliminate the exploitation and malpractice by these quacks. This can best be accomplished by educating the genuine medical practitioner about the diagnosis and management of ED, which they did not get to learn during their formal medical education.

While treating ED, one of the key skills one needs to have is 'counselling'; which involves being a good listener, giving adequate time and having empathy. I see a major lack of counselling skills in the medical fraternity in our country. This is because the formal training in 'counselling' and/or 'psychotherapy' is completely missing in our medical curriculum. This is true not only at the graduation or post-graduation levels, but also in the specialized training in M.D. psychiatry. As an insider, who has been formally associated with two prime medical colleges in Mumbai for over 45 years, from being a medical student in 1976 to now as a senior faculty, I have been a close witness to this unfortunate reality. Recognising this need, I started a counselling training facility in 1986 with my wife Dr. Minnu, who is a veteran in the field of Counselling Education & Training and Senior Psychotherapist at the 'Heart To Heart Counselling Centre'. At our institute we impart formal training to medical practitioners including psychiatrists, as well as medical students and allied healthcare professionals, in a wide range of counselling modalities.

I wish more and more medical practitioners take an interest in learning counselling along with a comprehensive knowledge about ED and other sexual dysfunctions, as only this can change the current scenario. This book is just one sincere step in that direction.

Dr. (Prof.) Rajan B. Bhonsle, M.D.

FOREWORD

Dr. Bharat Vatwani

To say that Erectile Dysfunction (ED) was my forte as a psychiatrist would be undermining the truth. In all honesty, it was the blind spot in my arsenal of knowledge that I had obtained during my academic career. My lack of knowledge on this particular subject was not something I was particularly proud of, but looking back - as far as ED is concerned, I'm afraid that perhaps the fault was not just with me but also lied in the fact that it was not easy to find material available in those days to read up on ED.

Whenever I sought to increase my knowledge on schizophrenia (which ultimately became my career focus) I would come across reams of papers and research written on it. ED remained woefully behind in being addressed as a separate topic of physical and psychological concern.

Sexology always addressed it as a whole without getting too specific. The common issue of ED was thus never addressed in isolation and in depth with a granular focus on its many facets. A tragedy of the scientific world. It goes without saying that the incidence of ED has always been high and it's an issue that has always been rampant in our country. It is this lacuna of knowledge which this dedicated book on ED addresses academically yet practically. The matter isn't delved into in a cursory manner. Dr. Rajan Bhonsle is not interested in simply skimming the surface.

This is a book of passionate research and it dares to dive deep into the subject in a lucid and minutely intrinsic manner. A treasure-trove for graduates and post graduates of literally all branches of medicine (since patients of ED can approach anyone to everyone - from cardiologists to sometimes even quacks) who wish to ameliorate the anguish, the stigma and the untold misery in their patients who approach them, often hesitantly, to find solutions and respite.

What is revealed to be an omnipotently prevalent problem in society must be given its due place in academic circles and this book has so deservingly achieved that.

Dr. Rajan Bhonsle has more than done justice to this complex subject.
A must-have and a must-read!

Dr. Bharat Vatwani,
M.D. (Psych Med)
Senior Consulting Psychiatrist
Founder, Shraddha Rehabilitation Foundation
Winner, Ramon Magsaysay Award (2018)

FOREWORD

Dr. Anup Ramani

Dr. Rajan Bhonsle is a nationally and internationally known name in the field of sexual medicine. The release of this book is timely! This is the first time that an Indian is analysing and addressing this rather common problem in India vis-a-vis Erectile Dysfunction (ED).

This is an often underdiagnosed issue. It is also a taboo subject in many circles. Erectile dysfunction is a crippling problem. It destroys marriages and self confidence in a man. It's a fairly complicated subject. Even a dedicated medical practitioner may find it difficult to diagnose the exact cause of the problem which leads to unsatisfied patients moving from doctor to doctor and sometimes even get exploited and misdirected by quacks in the hope of a remedy. Age is no bar and ED can afflict the young as well as a senior population.

The beauty of this book lies in its crystal-clear line of thinking on how to evaluate ED and the various treatment options available. The chapters systematically give the reader a deep insight into the world of ED. Treatments range from simple counselling to medications to surgery.

This book should be a compulsory addition in the libraries of every doctor who treats ED. I congratulate Dr. Rajan Bhonsle for writing this book and approaching such a difficult topic with much needed clarity and dignity. Dr. Rajan's knack for simplifying the complex is marvelous!

I would like to specially mention the "Frequently unasked questions" section of the book which covers almost every question a patient is likely to ask.

This is a landmark publication which will surely help budding doctors treating ED and even be a great resource guide for experts in the field.

Dr Anup Ramani, MS, MCh, DNB
Professor of Urology, Saifee Hospital Mumbai
Formerly, Joint Director, Uro-Oncology and Robotic Surgery,

Department of Urology, University of Minnesota, USA
Formerly, Fellow in Uro-Oncology, Cleveland Clinic foundation

Fellow in Robotic Surgery at IRCAD Hospital France.

FOREWORD

Dr. Kailash Gindodia

It is my absolute pleasure to write a review for a book written by my dear friend Dr. Rajan Bhonsle on the very hush-hush issue of Erectile Dysfunction (ED). This book offers up a detailed synopsis of ED and transcends the highly "google-able" explanation on the anatomy and physiology of an erection. It goes above and beyond that. It enumerates the various causes of ED and ways to diagnose and treat the issue while also beautifully illustrating that the most important sex organ is in fact the mind. The book calls out ED as the bio-psycho-social problem that it is and doesn't merely treat it as a physical issue. As most cases of ED are psychogenic this makes for an interesting exploration in addition to elucidating the detailed organic causes of the same.

Most men find it easier to talk to their doctor than to their partners about ED. This book should help these doctors effectively guide couples for a successful erection and happy sex life.

Evaluating a case of ED requires good history taking, a physical examination and certain lab-based investigations along with other specialised investigations like the rigiscan. The book explores such details. Regarding the treatment of ED, Dr. Rajan shares the good news that most types of ED can be addressed by treating the underlying physical or psychosocial problems that many physicians fail to point out or even understand. Dr. Rajan often quotes "what is good for your heart is good for your penis".

There are injectable / mechanical / surgical therapies illustrated in the book besides lifestyle modifications / oral therapies. This makes the book a holistic resource. A special chapter on Diabetes mellitus in ED is also included and I was impressed to read that as well. The book also helps encourage people to more open about consulting a sex therapist. It ends with a succinct chapter on frequently unanswered questions that perfectly completes the experience for the reader!

This book is a one-stop manual for any practitioner looking to educate himself or his patients on ED and I can happily say that this is a great investment for doctors and patients looking to learn more about a topic that's shrouded in mystery.

I wish Dr Rajan Bhonsle all the very best.

Dr. Kailash R Gindodia, M.S., Dip. Uro.
Professor and HOD Surgery, ACPM Medical College, Dhule

Author, KRG's Textbook of surgery, Handbook of Surgery & Mindmaps in Surgery

TABLE OF CONTENTS

Chapter 1
Mechanism of Erection

How does erection occur in male penis?

To understand how an erection (rigidity of the penis) occurs in men, we need to learn about the anatomy of the male penis.

The anatomy of a Penis

The penis is a cylindrical organ with the ability to be *flaccid* or *erect*. It provides a passage called the **urethra** for both the urine and semen. It can be a source of pleasure in response to sexual stimulation and is the organ that penetrates the vaginal canal during sexual intercourse.

The penis consists of a root, body (shaft) and glans (head). The head of the penis i.e., the glans (*glans penis*), is the part that is the most sensitive and has the most nerve endings (*neuro-receptors*). The ring or ridge of tissue that circles the lower edge of the glans is called the **corona**. The glans is covered by the foreskin (prepuce) in men who are not circumcised. A thin fold of skin is attached in a linear fashion underneath the glans in the midline. It is termed as the **frenulum**.

Normally, a man should be able to pull back his foreskin, enough to expose the whole of the "glans penis". This may either happen on its own on full erection or one may have to do it manually before penetration. Both ways it is normal and fine. If the retraction of the foreskin is not possible or is painful, then it is a medical condition known as **Phimosis**. This condition may require a minor surgery known as **Circumcision** which takes 20-30 minutes and is done under local anesthesia. Circumcision is a small surgery in which the foreskin covering the glans-penis is removed.

The penis is made up of three spongy tubes, each containing a sponge-like tissue that fills up with blood when the male is sexually excited. This is what causes an erection. The upper two tubes are called **Corpora Cavernosa** and the lower one is called **Corpus Spongiosum**. It is the corpus spongiosum through which the urethra passes out. All the three tubes are enveloped in a sheath called the **Tunica Albuginea**.

The corpus spongiosum and the two corpora cavernosa, each have an individual artery of their own that runs through their center. Arteries are the blood vessels that carry oxygenated blood from the heart to all parts of the body. The two corpora cavernosa are connected to each other in the middle of the penis, thus allowing blood to flow from one corpus cavernosa into the other. The veins that take the deoxygenated blood away from the corpora cavernosa back to our heart, run just beneath the tunica albuginea along the periphery of the corpora cavernosa. The veins are also different for the corpora cavernosa and corpus spongiosum.

Hemodynamics of Erection and Detumescence

When a man gets sexually aroused either by the sight, touch, sound or the thought of sex, the information travels from the brain to the nerve centers at the base of the spine, where the primary nerve fibers connect to the penis. His brain and his pelvic nerves release special pro-erectile chemicals called '**Neurotransmitters**'. These are the chemical messengers that signal the smooth muscles of the penile arteries to relax. The relaxation of smooth muscles in the penile arteries increases the blood flow in the corpora cavernosa. The corpora cavernosa has a spongy tissue. The way a sponge absorbs liquids into its air spaces and gets distended when submerged, the hollow spaces of the corpora cavernosa also get filled with blood in the same manner. This then gets distended with blood on sexual arousal as it causes increased blood flow into the penis. These hollow spaces are called **Sinusoids**. As the sinusoids get filled with blood and distend, they start compressing the veins against the tunica albuginea. The compression of the veins beneath the tunica albuginea prevents blood from leaving the penis, thus promoting full turgidity and maintenance of the erection.

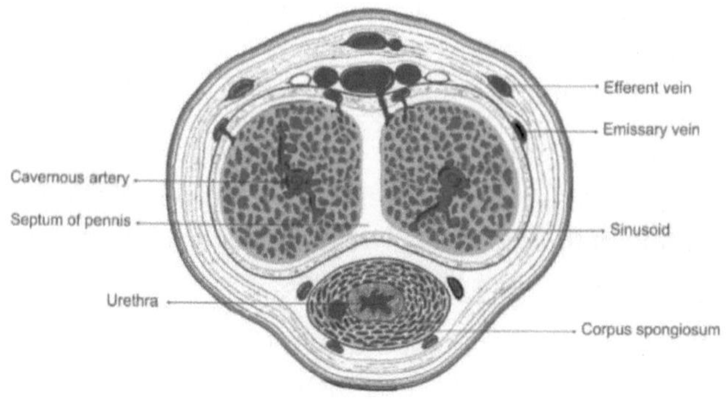

Once the sexual act is completed, the brain releases different chemicals that make the arteries in the penis to constrict, thus reducing the blood flow to the penis and allowing the veins to drain the blood out of the penis. These chemicals, that are responsible for the constriction of smooth muscle, can also get released when a person experiences stress, thus adversely affecting his erectile function.

A note on Neuroanatomy and Neurophysiology of Penile Erection

The innervation of the penis is both somatic (sensory and motor) as well as autonomic (sympathetic and parasympathetic).

The somato-sensory pathway originates at the sensory receptors in the glans penis, foreskin (prepuce) and within the corpus cavernosum. The somatic nerves are mainly responsible for sensation and the contraction of the ischiocavernosus and bulbocavernosus muscles. From the neurons in the spinal cord and peripheral ganglia, the sympathetic and parasympathetic nerves merge to form the cavernous nerves, which enter the corpora cavernosa and corpus spongiosum to affect the neurovascular events during erection and detumescence.

Depending on the nature and intensity of genital stimulation, many spinal reflexes can be elicited by stimulation of the genitalia. The bulbocavernosus reflex is the one such well identified reflexes.

This explains, that erections are not just something that occur only in the penis. For an erection to occur, it is necessary that there must be co-ordinated functioning of many systems in the body - the brain, the spinal cord, the pelvic nerves, the heart, the lungs, the arteries that supply blood to the penis and the veins that drain the blood from the penis.

The above explanation shows that the erectile process is a complex neurovascular event. The erectile function can be adversely affected when any disease process affects the brain, the pelvic nerves, the arteries of the penis, the veins in the penis, the tunica albuginea, or the actual erectile tissue within the corpora cavernosa.

Chapter 2
Defining Erectile Dysfunction

What is Erectile Dysfunction (ED)?

Previously, erectile dysfunction (ED) used to be commonly known as **'impotence'**. It is the persistent inability to achieve and/or sustain an erection for the satisfactory completion of sexual intercourse or activity. There are no uniform criteria defining how consistent the problem has to be and for what duration it must be present to be considered as an ED. The Diagnostic and Statistical Manual of Mental Disorders, (DSM-5) specifies a duration of at least 6 months in its definition of ED.

Looking carefully at the definition of ED, we can see that it is a 'subjective' definition. It means that the individual himself and/or his partner decides that his erections are not satisfactory. The definition is not an all-or-nothing one, as different men experience different degrees of erectile dysfunction.

It is necessary to understand that most men will experience this phenomenon at some point in their lives at least a few times. The situation plays out in the following manner – The man wants an erection, but quite unexpectedly is unable to get one. This is common and at times there is absolutely nothing to worry about. An occasional or situational erection problem does not mean that erectile dysfunction will become a chronic condition.

It is also important to note that the mind plays a very important role in getting an erection. A man unknowingly can sabotage his erection just by being anxious and worrying about his ability to perform, even in the absence of any physical problem.

'Performance Anxiety' is a very common problem in men. If a man is more focused on how well he is performing, rather than on enjoying the sensations in the sexual act, it may be difficult for him to attain or maintain an erection. This can become a vicious cycle, where the anxiety about having an erection becomes so severe that he is unable to have an erection and then this causes further anxiety. The way to remedy this problem is to learn to relax. The more the man relaxes and enjoys the experience of sexual touching, whether he has an erection or not, the more likely he will be able to get an erection and simply go with the flow.

Erectile dysfunction can become a problem only when it is persistent or frequent. An occasional failure to get an erection can be attributed to exhaustion, stress, fatigue, inadequate stimulation or even intoxication. Some men have a *'situational'* erectile inability. For example, they can get an erection when they are fantasizing and masturbating, but are unable to get one when they are with their partner. This usually means that the problem is primarily 'psychogenic'.

There are also men who are unable to get an erection in any situation, whether alone or with a partner. This usually suggests that the problem is predominantly organic (physical). Organic causes of erectile problems include diabetes, kidney disease, multiple sclerosis, Parkinson's disease, injuries to the spinal cord or brain, reactions to certain medications especially hypertension medications, antipsychotic and antidepressant drugs, chronic alcoholism, atherosclerosis or other vascular problems.

Erectile dysfunction is a 'symptom' and not a disease in and of itself. It could be a manifestation of an underlying medical condition. It is necessary to evaluate men with erectile dysfunction to identify the underlying disease process that is causing this problem. ED could also be a first or early symptom of an unidentified underlying medical condition that could cause further damage to the individual. Moreover, by treating the underlying disease processes, one can possibly prevent further progression of the erectile dysfunction.

Prevalence of Erectile Dysfunction

The first ever study that brought to light the prevalence of erectile dysfunction is the 'Massachusetts Male Ageing Study'. This study was conducted from 1987 to 1989 in 11 randomly selected cities and towns in the Boston metropolitan area and it included men between 40 to 70 years old.

This study revealed that 52% of men from the ages of 40 to 70 have some degree of erectile dysfunction. Out of those individuals, 10% reported complete erectile dysfunction, 25% reported moderate erectile dysfunction, and the rest 65% reported mild erectile dysfunction. The study also established that ED is progressively prevalent with age: approximately 40% of men are affected at the age of 40 and nearly 70% of men are affected at the age of 70.

The 'National Ambulatory Medical Care Survey' (NAMCS) conducted in 1985 in USA revealed that erectile dysfunction was associated with 525,000 outpatient office visits, while the 'National Hospital Discharge Survey' (NHDS) conducted in 1995 in USA reported that it accounted for more than 30,000 hospital admissions.

These studies showed that the prevalence rate of complete erectile dysfunction rises from 5% among men 40 years old to 15% among those 70 years old.

The occurrence of erectile dysfunction is found higher in men with certain medical conditions, such as diabetes mellitus, hyperlipidemia, thyroid disorders, hypertension, cardiovascular and neurological diseases and spinal cord afflictions.

More on Ageing and Erectile Dysfunction

As men age, they often notice the following -

- It takes 'longer' for them to achieve an erection. Men over 50 often take 2 to 3 times longer to attain an erection than younger men.
- They also notice that their erection may not be as firm or hard as it used to be in their younger years.
- The arousal alone may not be enough to get satisfactory rigidity without additional manual (tactile) stimulation.
- It also starts taking longer to climax.
- Ejaculation may or may not even occur, or it would happen with less force.
- The refractory period after ejaculation also increases with age. Many men above the age of 55 are unable to get another erection for 12 to 24 hours after ejaculation.

Failure to understand and accept these changes and to adapt to them may cause anguish, distress, frustration, anxiety and even depression, which may further complicate erectile function.

Age-related changes in sexual function occur due to the following physical changes –

- Decrease in the amount of smooth muscle in the penis.

- Atherosclerosis, loss of elasticity and hardening of blood vessels, suboptimal neurotransmission.
- The sensitivity of the penis can also diminish with age, thus it requires additional tactile stimulation to achieve an erection.
- Levels of free testosterone (the active from of testosterone) in the blood often decline.
- Chronic illnesses such as diabetes, hypertension, coronary artery disease etc are more common in the elderly, which further affect testosterone levels, nerve conduction and vascular response necessary for arousal and erection.

In cases of erectile dysfunction, the erections are either inadequate for penetration or they do not last long enough to complete the sexual act. It needs to be noted that the incidence of erectile dysfunction does increase with age, but still it need not be an expected process of ageing. Growing old as a rule is not always going to cause erectile dysfunction. Some men stay sexually functional into their 80s. How well one has maintained his health and fitness level is far more relevant, than a chronological age. Erectile dysfunction can be an early sign of a more serious health problem. Finding and treating the reason for erectile dysfunction is a vital first step, rather than attributing it to one's age.

Chapter 3
Causes of Erectile Dysfunction

Why men have difficulty in getting or sustaining erection?

Causes of Erectile dysfunction can be broadly classified into two etiologic categories:

- **Psychogenic** (Originating from the Mind/Psyche)

- **Organic** (Originating from the Body/Biology)

There was a time when most causes of erectile dysfunction were considered to be psychogenic for all age groups. However, current evidence suggests for those above the age of 40, up to 80 % of cases have an organic cause. For the age group younger than 40, up to 60-70 % of the cases have psychogenic causes.

There are some qualitative and clinically distinguishable differences between the erectile dysfunction induced by Psychogenic and Organic causes.

Psychogenic

- Acute onset
- Intermittent occurrence (situational, variability)
- Inability to sustain erection
- Reversible
- Good nocturnal and morning erection
- Response to phosphodiesterase type 5 (PDE 5) inhibitors is likely to be very good

Organic

- Gradual onset
- Persistently poor erectile response
- Inability to attain erection
- Often progressive
- Either weak or complete lack of nocturnal and morning erection
- Response to phosphodiesterase type 5 (PDE 5) inhibitors is uncertain
- Erection is better in the standing position than lying down (when the cause is a venous leak)

Organic causes of erectile dysfunction are further subdivided into four categories

- **Vasculogenic** (problems arising from the Cardio-vascular system)
- **Neurogenic** (problems arising from the Nervous system)
- **Hormonal** (problems arising from the Endocrine system)
- **Iatrogenic** (problems arising from medical intervention or treatment)

While the above classifications are made for the sake of clarity, there is invariably a combination of more than one cause. Practically, all organic causes invariably have a superadded Psychogenic cause to make a combined aetiology.

Often, even after successfully treating the organic cause, the patient continues to experience a significant degree of erectile difficulty due to an unresolved or inadequately addressed coexisting psychogenic component. This makes it obvious that a treating clinician needs to have adequate training and experience in Counselling skills and/or Psychotherapeutic techniques such as Rational Emotive Behaviour Therapy (REBT), Transactional Analysis (TA) along with Rogerian client-centred approach such as Robert Carkhuff model. Lack of proper training in Counselling, often leaves the most competent physicians or surgeons ineffective to treat cases of erectile dysfunction completely.

Psychogenic Causes of Erectile Dysfunction

For a normal sexual activity, the mind and body need to work together. Psychological, emotional or relationship problems are known to adversely affect every aspect of the sexual activity – desire, erection and even ejaculation.

Psychogenic causes of erectile dysfunction can further be divided into three categories:

- **Relational** (When the cause of ED is in the status of relationship with the sex partner e.g. attraction, expectations, presumptions, biases, conflicts, arising out of emotional conflicts in relationship with a sex partner)

- **Non-Relational** (When the cause of ED is unrelated to the partner)

- **Situational** (When the cause of ED lies in the situation, unrelated to the partner)

Let us explore the above three categories of psychogenic ED

Relational causes of Psychogenic ED

(When the cause of ED is in the status of relationship with sex partner)

Disturbed relationship often results into loss of attraction and interest in sex causing psychogenic ED.

- **Lack or loss of physical attraction for the partner:** This can happen due to specific or rigid expectations of physical attributes in a partner (e.g. certain shape and size of breasts, hips, legs etc), specific and/or rigid expectations of hygiene standards in the partner, dressing and grooming, and even the degree and manner in which the 'interest in sex' is either expressed or not expressed by the partner. Certain mannerisms, gestures and styles of communication of the partner can also result into lack or loss of sexual attraction for the partner.

- **Conflicts with the partner:** Misunderstandings, difference of opinion, mismatching of values, ideas and lifestyle choices, insults, put downs, abusive verbal exchange, physical abuse, extramarital affairs, addictions, personality disorders, mental instability, mood and thought disorders etc invariably result in a disturbed relationship causing loss of sexual attraction for each other.

- **Real or imaginary fear of the partner's expectations, reactions or responses:** Fear, imagination or anticipation of partner's real or projected expectation can cause heightened anxiety in some men resulting into psychogenic ED. E.g. fear of the partner's actual or anticipated reaction towards one's penis size or the 'stamina' to last or the ability to satisfy the partner

Besides these, prolonged disconnect with the partner due to the nature of work/job or travel, interest in some other partner, lack of coordination of time for intimacy, lack of communication with the partner about one's sexual expectations, preoccupation with sexual fantasy are also some additional relational causes of psychogenic ED.

Non-Relational causes of Psychogenic ED

(When the cause of ED is unrelated to the partner or the status of relationship with the partner)

Many psychological and emotional disturbances arise out of reasons that have nothing to do with the partner or the status of relationship between the two. These disturbances arise from everyday life issues related to work, money, career, reputation, self-esteem, past experiences, misinformation and health. Even though these causes are no way linked with the partner, they affect the sexual desire and thus result into psychogenic ED.

- Lack of self-esteem and body image issues
- Feeling nervous about or self-conscious about sex
- Loss of job, business or professional reputation
- Work stress due to excessive work load, dominating and exploitative superiors, inconsiderate or uncooperative subordinates, power politics, groupism, change of work profile, diminishing resources etc
- Financial loss due to mistakes, fraud, wrong decisions, bad deals, cheating, stock market downturn etc
- Illness or death of a close family member, friend or neighbour
- Stress from social, cultural or religious conflicts
- Prior traumatic sexual experience such as sexual abuse, rape, molestation etc
- Fear of unwanted pregnancy
- Religious beliefs, guilt or inhibitions
- Litigations, allegations, loss of reputation and respect

- Failure or fear of failure in competitive examination, job interview etc

- Impending medical test reports

While a person is going through any of the above issues, a supportive and sympathetic partner can play a very important role in the recovery.

On the other hand, a critical, nagging, blaming, dismissive spouse can add further stress resulting into more severe form of psychogenic ED. In such a situation, relational and non-relational issues can not just add up but multiply the severity and gravity of psychogenic ED.

Situational causes of Psychogenic ED

While the relationship and mutual attraction in partners may be in place or could even be thriving, there may not be any other major non-relational issue in life. However certain situations, times and settings can still cause psychogenic ED.

- **Lack of privacy** Small or crowded homes with no provision for privacy

- **Time constraints** due to mismatching job timings, pressure of deadlines, bad time management etc

- **Weather constraints** such as very low or very high temperature

- **Space constraints** such as small sized bed, uncomfortable bedding, noisy, smelly or unclean bed or room etc

- **Responsibility constraints** due to reasons such as illness of a close one like an old parent or a child or a pet that needs constant attention

Situational causes are often temporary (not long lasting) and positively rectifiable. All it requires is a coordinated strategy and adequate efforts to minimise or rectify the situational factor. An experienced sex counsellor or a trained therapist can offer a wide range of practical suggestions to counter situational factors, as professionally they often deal with similar situations with other clients. Thus, they may be consulted to ideate, to get tips and suggestions to take care of a situational cause of ED.

How Psychogenic causes affect the mechanism of an erection

Psychogenic causes make a person hesitate, resist or block sexual thoughts and feelings, thus not allowing the whole neuro-vascular mechanism of an erection to kick-in and get activated. They consciously or unconsciously tend to block the very first sexual impulses at the psychological (thoughts and feelings) level.

However, there are also actual physiological changes that take place in the body, secondary to psychological causes that proactively inhibit arousal and erection. These changes are explained here for those with academic interest.

Activation of Sympathetic nervous system.

An erection is a carefully coordinated chain of events controlled by our nervous system. The male sexual response shows a dynamic balance between exciting and inhibiting forces of the 'Autonomic Nervous System' within the penis and all through the nervous system. The Autonomic Nervous System has two components – Sympathetic and Parasympathetic. The sympathetic component tends to inhibit erections, whereas the parasympathetic system encourages sexual excitement.

When a man feels stressful, his amygdala (an area of the brain that contributes to emotional processing) starts sending a 'distress signal' to the hypothalamus. Hypothalamus is the part of the brain that functions like a command center. It communicates with the rest of the body through the nervous system. Hypothalamus activates the sympathetic nervous system by sending signals to the adrenal glands through the autonomic nerves. Adrenal glands quickly respond by pumping the hormone 'adrenaline' into the bloodstream. This causes suppression of arousal as well as erection.

Organic causes of Erectile Dysfunction

When the cause of erectile dysfunction is in the biology (physical body) of the person, it is termed as **Organic Erectile Dysfunction**. Organic causes are generally the result of an underlying medical condition affecting either the blood vessels or the nerves supplying the penis.

Before we look into the organic causes of erectile dysfunction, let us look at some of the known 'risk factors' that make a person vulnerable to develop organic erectile dysfunction.

- Obesity
- Smoking
- Alcohol abuse
- Age - Being over 50
- Hypertension *(high blood pressure)*

- Diabetes mellitus *(high blood sugar level)*
- Liver conditions *(suboptimal functioning of liver)*
- Hyperlipidaemia *(High Cholesterol and Triglycerides)*
- Thyroid Problems *(Hypothyroidism and Hyperthyroidism)*
- Sedentary lifestyle *(Lack of exercise and low level of physical activity)*

Many of the above are not only the risk factors or predisposing factors, but can also become the 'primary cause' of erectile dysfunction at a later date. Younger patients with one or many of these predisposing factors may not be experiencing erectile dysfunction currently, however in times to come they will certainly encounter erectile dysfunction either much earlier or in much more severe and irreversible form than the same-age population. More the risk factors, earlier and severer will be the nature of erectile dysfunction. Treatment also becomes more complex, less effective and prolonged in nature with lower success rate when there are a greater number of risk factors.

Even though erectile dysfunction becomes more common as men age, it does not mean as a rule 'growing old' is going to cause it. There are men who stay sexually functional even into their 80s. Moreover, erectile dysfunction can be treated at any age.

It is necessary to remember that erectile dysfunction can be the first sign or one of the early signs of a more serious health problem. Thus, finding and treating the reason for erectile dysfunction is an important and imperative first step.

Organic causes are subdivided into four categories

- **Vasculogenic** (arising from Cardio-vascular system problems)
- **Neurogenic** (arising from Nervous system problems)
- **Hormonal** (arising from Endocrine system problems)
- **Iatrogenic** (arising from medical intervention or treatment)

Vasculogenic Erectile Dysfunction

Erection is a neurovascular event. Blood vessels play a very vital role in the mechanism of erection. From a vascular viewpoint, any disease process that can affect our arteries can also affect the arteries that supply blood to the penis.

Atherosclerosis

Atherosclerosis is a process in which plaque builds up inside our arteries and start narrowing our arteries. This starts compromising the 'blood flow' through narrowed arteries. As blood flow is the mandatory aspect of erectile process, when atherosclerosis starts obstructing and compromising the blood flow through arteries that supply penis, it leads to erectile dysfunction. Plaques are made up of fat, cholesterol, calcium, and some other substances in the blood. In the extreme form of atherosclerosis plaque can completely block the artery. This is found in

- Coronary artery diseases (Angina pectoris or Myocardial infarction)
- Cerebrovascular diseases (transient ischemic attack or stroke)
- Peripheral vascular disease (PVD) – It is a blood circulation disorder that causes the blood vessels outside of your heart and brain to narrow, block, or spasm. Besides arteriosclerosis, hardening of the

peripheral arteries or spasms of blood vessel can also cause PVD.

Hypertension (High blood pressure)

High blood pressure damages the lining of arteries causing them to become thicker, to harden and narrow. This keeps the arteries that carry blood into the penis from dilating the way they are supposed to. This **can** restrict the blood flow to your penis, which may then cause erectile dysfunction.

Hyperlipidaemia (High cholesterol and triglycerides)

Previously the association between hyperlipidemia and erectile dysfunction was entirely attributed to atherosclerosis process in the entire hypogastric-cavernosal arterial bed, resulting into a subsequent insufficiency in penile arterial inflow.

Now it is also discovered that hyperlipidemia adversely affects the endothelial cells and smooth muscles of the penis and even the peripheral nerves, which further contributes to erectile difficulties.

It is also found in more recent researches that high cholesterol in particular can make the body more difficult to produce the chemicals that are necessary to produce an erection. High cholesterol hampers the body's ability to release 'nitric oxide' into the bloodstream. This prevents the proper relaxation of penile tissues to have engorgement of blood into penis to produce erection.

Arterial damage due to trauma

Trauma to pelvic or perineal vasculature due to reasons such as vehicular accident, fall or direct injury to the penis can also cause vasculogenic erectile dysfunction in a person. This greatly depends on which blood vessels are damaged and to what extent.

Venous Leak

The penis is expected to get filled with blood to maintain an erection. If the veins are unable to hold on to this engorged blood during an erection, a man will lose the erection. This is called **Caverno-Venous leakage**, simply known as a **Venous Leak.** It is the inability to sustain an erection in the presence of adequate arterial blood flow through the cavernosal arteries of the penis. The weakness lies in the undue drainage of veins in the cavernosal tissue of the penis, which weakens normal erectile function.

This is seen as the curable cause of erectile dysfunction. Surgical approach involves ligation of all identified leaking veins.

More on Venous Leak

'Cavernosography with Cavernosometry' is the diagnostic reference standard for the diagnosis of venous leak. This technique measures outflow resistance without the need for adequate arterial inflow. It also helps mapping the sites of leakage. However, Cavernosography is done only if surgical venous ligation is planned.

Surgical intervention for venous leak has a rather low success rate and even its effectiveness is found short-lived. However, it being relatively minor and a safe surgical procedure, and if it is also the treatment of choice, it can be undertaken with informed consent by a skilled surgeon. In cases of younger patients with site-specific congenital, post-inflammatory or post-traumatic venous leaks, vein ligation can certainly be considered. An alternative treatment option is 'coil embolization' via a direct approach using a draining vein.

The choice of procedure offered should be decided on available facilities including infrastructure, the experience and preference of the treating expert, and the basis of the site, nature, and size of the leak.

More recently 3D-CT cavernosography has emerged as an advanced diagnostic option. It provides high-resolution images of venous leakage from any angle. The images taken by 3D-CT cavernosography are far more helpful to know the anatomical study of the human penile venous system, for the diagnosis of corporal veno-occlusive dysfunction, which can further help to plan superior treatment strategies in treating erectile dysfunction due to venous leak.

Of late, penile venous surgery with *crural ligation* for venous leakage has shown very good long-term results and higher patient satisfaction. Young patients with normal penile arterial system and no other risk factors (such as diabetes, hypertension, obesity etc.) have a better chance to enhance their erection quality and duration post-operatively.

Neurogenic Erectile Dysfunction

Erection is a neurovascular event. Nervous system plays a very pivotal role in the mechanism of erection. A wide range of neurological condition can cause erectile dysfunction.

Long spread tracts of the central nervous system, starting from cerebral cortex to the sacral spinal cord require to be intact for the normal physiological sexual function. Sexual arousal takes place due to a wide range of perceived as well as imagined stimuli and responses are achieved by conduction of these impulses down the spinal cord and through the peripheral and autonomic nervous system to the penis.

Any condition that hampers or obstructs this process can cause neurogenic erectile dysfunction. Following is the list of neurologic Conditions that cause erectile dysfunction.

- Lumbo-Sacral Spine diseases such as Intervertebral Disc prolapse or herniation, disc degeneration, Spondylolisthesis, Spina bifida, Spinal canal stenosis, lesions affecting the parasympathetic innervation by S2–S4 roots etc

- Spinal cord injury or a mass

- Cauda equina lesions. The collection of nerves at the end of the spinal cord is known as the cauda equina. When the nerve roots of the cauda equina are compressed or damaged, it causes disruption of motor and sensory functions and also results into neurogenic erectile dysfunction

- Temporal lobe epilepsy

- Parkinson's disease

- Multiple Sclerosis

- Alzheimer's disease

- Pituitary disease such as pituitary adenoma

- Stroke

- Radiation therapy

- Surgical procedures, such as radical prostatectomy i.e. a prostate removal surgery can cause injury to the pelvic nerves resulting into neurogenic erectile dysfunction. The incidence of erectile dysfunction after radical prostatectomy depends on whether a "nerve-sparing" surgical procedure was performed or not. Reported rates of erectile dysfunction after bilateral nerve-sparing radical prostatectomy range from 18 to 82%.

Hormone induced Erectile Dysfunction

Hormones are chemical messengers. They regulate countless bodily functions. When hormone levels get disturbed, symptoms, imbalances and malfunctions follow soon. Erectile dysfunction is one such potential problem that can be caused by a hormonal imbalance.

Hormones, such as testosterone, prolactin, or thyroid, are particularly known for causing erectile dysfunction.

The list of hormonal conditions that are commonly associated with erectile dysfunction is given below:

- **Hypogonadism** *(lower testosterone secretion)*
- **Diabetes Mellitus** *(High blood sugar level)*
- **Hyperthyroidism** *(overactive thyroid gland)*
- **Hypothyroidism** *(underactive thyroid gland)*
- **Hyperprolactinemia** *(increased prolactin secretion by Pituitary gland)*
- **Anabolic steroid abuse**, found in body builders

Hypogonadism

Hypogonadism is also known as 'testosterone deficiency'. It is a failure of the testes to produce the male sex hormone testosterone, sperm, or both.

Testosterone is the principal biological determinant of the 'sex drive' in both men and women. Testosterone plays many roles in the human body. In men, testosterone is responsible for the development and maintenance of the primary sexual characteristics as well as secondary sexual characteristics. It is also responsible for the sex drive (libido) and helps us to have an erection. Low testosterone levels can result in erectile dysfunction.

There is a separate dedicated chapter on Hypogonadism in this book, that explains hypogonadism in detail.

Diabetes Mellitus

To get an erection, a man needs healthy blood vessels, nerves, testosterone hormones, and a desire for sex. Diabetes can damage the blood vessels and nerves that are connected with an erection. Therefore, even if a person has normal testosterone level and has the desire to have sex, he may still not be able to attain a firm erection.

It is estimated that about 35% to 75% of men with diabetes mellitus experience some degree of erectile dysfunction during their lifetime. They also tend to develop erectile dysfunction about 10 to 15 years earlier than those without diabetes.

There is a separate dedicated chapter on 'Diabetes Mellitus and Erectile Dysfunction' in this book, that explains relationship of diabetes and erection in detail.

Hypothyroidism and Hyperthyroidism

Hypothyroidism occurs when the thyroid gland does not produce adequate thyroid hormones. Hyperthyroidism refers to an overactive thyroid, when the gland produces too much thyroid hormones. Both hypothyroidism as well as hyperthyroidism can affect a man's ability to achieve erections.

The Journal of Clinical Endocrinology published a research report in 2008, which says that 79% of the 71 men with thyroid problems had some degree of erectile dysfunction. It was found more common in men with hypothyroidism as compared to men with hyperthyroidism. However, an effective treatment for both these conditions is available and can significantly correct erection problems.

Hyperprolactinemia

Prolactin is a hormone produced in the pituitary gland, named originally after its function to promote milk production (Pro-lactation). It helps in stimulating and maintaining production of breast milk.

Hyperprolactinemia describes an excess of prolactin hormone in a person's body. Hyperprolactinemia is known for inducing hypogonadism (low level of Testosterone). The excess production of prolactin in the pituitary gland interferes with the secretion of gonadotropin-releasing hormone (GnRH), resulting in a decreased testosterone level, thus causing erectile dysfunction.

Hyperprolactinemia is invariably caused by a benign pituitary tumor - Prolactinoma. The large number of patients with hyperprolactinemia can be effectively treated using dopamine agonist drugs such as Bromocriptine and Cabergoline; however, in advanced cases even surgery can be done.

Anabolic Steroid Abuse

Supra-physiologic anabolic-androgenic steroid (AAS), briefly referred as steroids or Anabolic steroids are synthetic versions of the male hormone testosterone. Some misguided body builders and athletes abuse them to build muscles and to increase athletic performance and strength. Use of anabolic steroids is legally banned worldwide by all major international sports bodies.

Anabolic steroids provide synthetic testosterone to the body, which can cause the body itself to stop producing natural testosterone (hypogonadism). The body feels that testosterone is supplied from other sources, so it stops producing its own natural testosterone. This is the foremost reason why men experience erectile dysfunction when they are on anabolic steroids. Prolonged use of anabolic steroids causes shrinkage of testicles (testicular atrophy) and also a reduced sperm count (Oligospermia). Anabolic steroids can also increase the risk of developing testicular cancer, especially when they are used in combination with insulin-like growth factor.

Iatrogenic

Iatrogenic disorders are those arising from a medical treatment or intervention. It occurs either as a side effect or an outcome of a medical procedure, manoeuvre or surgery. This can happen either out of no choice when benefits of treatment are assessed or guessed to be more beneficial than the possible side effect.

Erectile dysfunction (ED) can be Iatrogenic. It is known to be a common side effect of a number of prescription drugs. While these medications may control or treat a disease, but in the process of doing so they can affect either hormones, nerves or blood vessels, resulting either in erectile dysfunction or by increasing the risk of ED.

Common group of medications that can cause ED as a potential side effect:

- Hormones
- Tranquilizers
- Antipsychotics
- Antihistamines
- Antidepressants
- Muscle relaxants

- Prostate cancer drugs
- H2-receptor antagonists
- Anti-seizure medications
- Parkinson's disease drugs
- Chemotherapy medications
- Nonsteroidal anti-inflammatory drugs
- Antiandrogens (androgen antagonists)
- Antihypertensives (high blood pressure drugs)
- Antiarrhythmics (drug for irregular heart action)
- Diuretics (medications that cause increase urine flow)

If patient is having problems achieving or maintaining an erection, it may be good idea take a look at the medicines that he is taking.

The list of drugs that may cause erectile dysfunction

1. **Drugs for high blood pressure (Antihypertensives) and Diuretics**

- Atenolol
- Bumetanide
- Captopril
- Chlorthalidone
- Clonidine
- Enalapril
- Furosemide
- Guanfacine
- Hydralazine
- Hydrochlorothiazide
- Labetalol
- Methyldopa
- Metoprolol
- Nifedipine
- Propranolol

- Phenoxybenzamine
- Spironolactone
- Triamterene
- Verapamil

2. Anti-anxiety drugs, Anti-depressants, and Anti-epileptic drugs

- Amitriptyline
- Amoxipine
- Buspirone
- Clomipramine
- Chlordiazepoxide
- Clorazepate
- Desipramine
- Diazepam
- Doxepin
- Fluoxetine
- Imipramine
- Isocarboxazid
- Lorazepam
- Nortriptyline
- Oxazepam
- Phenytoin
- Phenelzine
- Sertraline
- Tranylcypromine

3. Anti-Histamines

- Dimehydrinate
- Diphenhydramine
- Hydroxyzine
- Meclizine
- Promethazine

4. Parkinson's disease medications

- Benztropine
- Biperiden
- Bromocriptine
- Levodopa
- Procyclidine
- Trihexyphenidyl

5. Non-steroidal Anti-Inflammatory drugs

- Indomethacin
- Naproxen

6. Muscle relaxants

- Cyclobenzaprine
- Orphenadrine

7. Histamine H2-receptor antagonists

- Cimetidine
- Nizatidine
- Ranitidine

There are many more drugs that affect libido, arousal and erection, besides the list given above.

If a patient experiences ED and thinks that it may be a result of medication, he should not stop taking the drug without first consulting his doctor. If the problem persists, the doctor may be able to prescribe a different medication.

Other medical interventions that can cause ED

Besides medications that adversely affect erectile function, there are some other medical interventions that can also cause erectile dysfunction. Some such interventions are listed below:

- **Orchidectomy surgery**
- **Prostate surgery**
- **Radical pelvic surgery**

Generally, the damage that occurs during these above-mentioned procedures is primarily neurogenic in nature (cavernous nerve injury) but accessory pudendal artery injury can also contribute to the damage.

- **Hemodialysis** for renal (kidney) failure

Erectile dysfunction occurs in a large number (82%) of men on hemodialysis for renal (kidney) failure. Men on hemodialysis are more likely to experience erectile dysfunction if they are older, if they have diabetes mellitus, and if they do not use medications called Angiotensin Converting Enzyme (ACE) inhibitors. The cause of the erectile dysfunction is probably multifactorial; it may be partly related to the medical condition that caused the renal failure (e.g. diabetes mellitus), but it also may be related to hormonal changes that occur with dialysis. Dialysis patients have lower testosterone levels and may have high prolactin levels. In addition, dialysis lowers zinc levels and may cause overactivity of the parathyroid gland (hyperparathyroidism).

Chapter 4
Diagnosis of Erectile Dysfunction

Investigating and Evaluating Erectile Dysfunction

The diagnosis and primary evaluation of erectile dysfunction requires :

- **History taking**
- **Physical examination**
- **Investigations** (Laboratory tests and other specialized investigations)

History Taking

The first and the foremost step in evaluating erectile dysfunction is a detailed history taking. While taking the history, it is necessary to first establish that the problem truly is erectile dysfunction and not some other form of sexual dysfunction. Very often, any form of sexual difficulty to initiate, execute and complete the act of sexual intercourse is collectively referred as erectile dysfunction by the patient. Where as in reality there are several causes besides erectile dysfunction that can come in the way of initiating or completing the act of intercourse. A very common example of this is 'premature ejaculation'.

The history also helps the clinician to distinguish between the organic and the psychogenic causes of erectile dysfunction. E.g. If a man gives a history such as "no sexual difficulty until last night," the problem is most likely related to performance anxiety, situational or psychological problem.

It is necessary to explore the onset, duration and progression of the problem. E.g., If the inability to hold on to an erection or the loss of erection (detumescence) 'after penetration' is an occasional experience, it is most likely due to anxiety. However, if it is happening persistently, every time, even in the most unanxious times, then it is suggestive of 'vascular steel syndrome'. In the vascular steel syndrome, blood gets redirected from the distended corpora cavernosae to meet the oxygen requirements of the thrusting pelvis.

Questions need to be asked regarding the presence or absence of nocturnal or morning erections as well as about the ability to masturbate and frequency of masturbation. Complete loss of nocturnal or morning erections and the persistent inability to masturbate at any time are often signs of vascular or neurological disease.

A personal history about risk factors such as smoking, alcohol abuse, hypertension, past illnesses, past trauma or surgery, and endocrinal problems such as hypo or hyperthyroidism and diabetes is also very important.

The knowledge of the patient's current and past medications for any other health issue or illness is very important. Many necessary and effective medications given for other health issues such as hypertension, dyslipidaemia, depression, epilepsy etc are known to cause a loss of sexual desire and difficulty with erection as a side effect.

Finally, history of any psychological issues, any psychiatric problems is also very important. It helps the clinician to identify and trace psychological, emotional and relational issues as causative factors such as marital discord, interpersonal conflicts, adjustment issues, stress, depression and anxiety.

History taking involves number of direct and personal questions about the medical, social and sexual background of a patient. The list of such questions is given below. Some of these questions might be embarrassing and uncomfortable, however the patient needs to answer them as honestly as possible, as this probably could be the most significant part of the diagnostic process. It helps the treating clinician to identify predisposing factors for psychogenic as well as organic erectile dysfunction.

List of questions that need to be asked by a clinician during history taking to evaluate the cause and the severity of the erectile dysfunction:

- How long have you been experiencing erectile dysfunction?
- Was the onset abrupt or gradual?
- Is the problem constant or intermittent?
- Is it progressively deteriorating your erection quality and duration?
- Can you recollect any precipitating event when you first experienced it?
- Do you get your erection hard enough to be able to have vaginal penetration?
- Does your erection last long enough for completion of sexual act to the satisfaction of you and your partner?
- Does it occur only during partner sex or even during masturbation?
- Does it occur with only one particular partner or with any other partner? (in case of multiple partners)
- Are you able to achieve erection with a certain fantasy or with certain type of stimulation?
- Do you notice nocturnal or morning erection?
- Is there any penile curving or pain associated with your erection?
- Do you have any urinary complaints?
- Are you on any medication for prostate problem?

- When did you have your last medical check-up done? And what was the reason?
- Are you diabetic or hypertensive?
- Are you on any regular medications for any other health issue?
- Have you had any major illness or surgery in the past?
- Do you ride a bicycle regularly? And if so, since how long and how often?
- Are you taking any treatment for hair fall (Alopecia)?
- Have you had any spinal or pelvic injury either due to a vehicular accident or a fall?
- Do you smoke? And if so, since how long? How many cigarettes do you smoke every day?
- Do you drink alcohol? and if so, how often and how much?
- Do you use any recreational drug?
- Do you feel stressed out, anxious or depressed either due to erectile dysfunction or due to any other cause?
- Is your partner eager and interested in participating in your treatment and work on improving your sexual relationship?

Some sexologists ask patient to complete following questionnaire –

- The International Index of Erectile Function (IIEF) or
- The Brief Sexual Health Inventory for Men (SHIM)

The SHIM is the condensed version of IIEF with only five questions.

These questionnaires can also be helpful in assessing the ED and can also help to assess patient's response to therapies.

Physical Examination

A thorough physical examination involves looking for
clinical signs of several disorders that may be causing the
erectile dysfunction in the patient - such as hypertension,
cardiovascular disease, neurological problems,
peripheral vascular disease, renal or liver disease, thyroid
problems etc.

In the physical examination the clinician looks for :

- **Head and neck**, to rule out icterus (yellow sclera),
  anemia, thyroid enlargement and tenderness, and
  also any enlarged lymph nodes.
- **Visual field defects**, to rule out prolactinoma or
  pituitary mass.
- **Pulse and blood pressure**, to determine whether
  there might be a cardio-vascular problem.
- **Chest**, to see how well lungs and heart are
  functioning and to look for Gynecomastia (tender or
  enlarged breasts in males), which is indicative of
  pituitary problem.
- **Abdomen**, examined by inspection and palpation to
  rule out enlarged liver, spleen or kidneys, any
  abdominal masses, rigidity, guarding or tenderness.
- **Genitalia,** examined by inspection and palpation to
  see any penile deformity, curvature, presence of
  plaques, presence and elasticity of foreskin and
  whether it can be retracted to expose the glans penis
  to rule of any phimosis, look for hygiene status of
  glans penis, presence of smegma or signs of Balanitis
  (inflammation of the glans).

  It is also necessary to check the testes to make sure
  that both are present, are of normal size and
  consistency, and have no masses, any presence of

Hydrocele (collection of fluid in the scrotum), Varicocele (enlargement of the veins within scrotum), to look for secondary sexual characteristics, such as presence of pubic hair, normal growth of penis and testes.

- **Femoral pulse**, **femoral bruits, Dorsalis pedis pulse** (pulses in feet), to rule out any peripheral vascular disease.
- **Penile sensation, reflexes, and rectal tone**. This involves checking the bulbocavernosus reflex by inserting a finger in the rectum, squeezing the tip of penis, and noting a contraction of the anus at time of squeezing penis. If this reflex is absent, it is indicative of a problem in the pelvis. Digital rectal examination also helps to make prostate assessment.
- **Sacral and perineal neurological exam** can also be done to assess autonomic function.

While the entire battery of physical examination pointers is given above, the treating clinician is at a liberty to select those examinations which he finds more relevant and necessary for the case they are treating. The choice and the order of examination is often decided by the clinician on the basis of his assessment, experience and expertise.

Laboratory tests

The laboratory evaluation of the patient is the third and an equally important step to diagnose and plan the treatment of erectile dysfunction. An exhaustive list of laboratory tests is given below with brief rationale behind doing each test. More elaborate significance of these tests is described in this book at various places where the explanation is relevant and useful.

Following set of laboratory tests can be advised:

1. **Complete Blood Count (CBC):** This test helps the clinician to screen and evaluate a patient's overall health and also to detect, confirm and monitor a wide range of disorders.

2. **Erythrocyte Sedimentation Rate (ESR):** This test helps clinician to identify and measure inflammation causing conditions (infections, autoimmune diseases and cancers) anywhere in our body.

3. **Blood Sugar - Fasting and Post-prandial with Urine Sugar**: Estimation of Blood sugar is necessary to diagnose, estimate and monitor Diabetes, which is one of the prominent and treatable causes of ED.

4. **Liver Function Tests (Liver Profile):** It is a group of blood tests that show how well the liver is working. These tests measure the levels of certain enzymes, proteins and bilirubin in blood which help diagnose and monitor liver damage.

   - *Patients with liver disease are known to present with clinical features of hypogonadism, with or without testicular atrophy; such as decreased libido, ED and infertility. The severity of liver cirrhosis often correlates with the degree of ED.*

   - *Nonalcoholic fatty liver disease (NAFLD) is known as the hepatic manifestation of Metabolic Syndrome (MetS). The relation between metabolic syndrome (MetS) and ED is well known.*

   - *ED is also extremely common among men with cirrhosis of the liver, affecting almost 50% of men who develop cirrhosis.*

5. **Kidney Function Tests (Renal Profile):** It is a group of tests that help in identifying the presence of renal disease, determining the progression of renal disease

and monitoring the response to treatment. Men with malfunctioning kidneys experience variety of sexual problems such as loss of sex drive and ED. This happens due to a number of reasons.

- *The renin-angiotensin-aldosterone system of the kidneys regulates our blood pressure by managing blood volume. In cases of kidney damage, this mechanism gets adversely affected, thus causing renal hypertension. High blood pressure in turn can cause arteries around the kidneys to weaken, narrow or harden, thus not being able to deliver enough blood to the kidneys, causing further renal damage. This works like a vicious cycle.*

- *People with Renal Hypertension are often put on antihypertensive drugs which have a side effect of ED.*

- *Kidney patients often have narrowed blood vessels all over their body, including those vessels supplying to the penis. This decreases the blood supply to the penis, thus making it difficult to get an erection.*

- *It is also found that in men with kidney failure, they develop venous leak (blood leaks back out of the penis), causing loss of erection.*

- *The levels of testosterone is often found either higher or lower in those with kidney failure as compared to normal people of the same age.*

6. **Lipid Profile:** It is a panel of blood tests that helps as a primary screening tool for abnormalities in lipids, such as cholesterol and triglycerides. The results of this test can approximately estimate risks for

cardiovascular disease, certain forms of pancreatitis, and some other diseases.

- *Increased cholesterol level in the bloodstream creates atherosclerosis (arterial plaques) that hampers and blocks blood flow. This leads to inadequate circulation of blood throughout the body including the penis and genital area. As a result, erection problem starts occurring.*

- *Hyperlipidemia at an early stage can affect the endothelial cells, smooth muscles of the penis and even the peripheral nerves that are necessary for penile erection.*

- *High cholesterol adversely affects the body's ability to release 'nitric oxide' into the bloodstream. This hinders the proper relaxation of penile tissues to bring about erectile engorgement.*

- *High cholesterol limits blood flow to the testicles. As a result, can damage their ability to produce testosterone.*

7. **Serum Testosterone – Total and Free:** This test measures the level of testosterone in the blood. Testosterone is the main sex hormone (androgen) in men, produced mainly by the testicles, and is responsible for the sexual desire (libido) and development of secondary sexual characteristics in males. The testosterone level fluctuates throughout the day and is highest in the morning; thus it is advisable to have the testosterone level checked always in the morning. There are several reasons why testosterone level is tested during the evaluation of ED.

- *To assess whether testosterone supplement can improve low libido, which might be the cause of the ED. If there is a decrease in your libido and the testosterone level is found low, then testosterone supplement can improve your libido. This may not always resolve the ED if there are more than one causes of ED.*

- *In some men with liver disease, the total testosterone level may be low, but the 'free' testosterone level (the active form of testosterone) is normal. If the testosterone level is low, then a prolactin level should be checked to rule out a pituitary adenoma.*

- *A benign pituitary tumor (adenoma) can suppress testosterone production and cause decreased libido and ED. These tumors are treatable effectively, and the loss of libido and ED are potentially reversible.*

8. **Sex Hormone Binding Globulin (SHBG):** This test measures the level of Sex Hormone Binding Globulin (SHBG) in our blood. SHBG is a protein made by our liver. After the testosterone is produced, most of it binds with SHBG. Testosterone in this bound state is not available for our cells to use. Only 1-2 per cent of the total production of testosterone is the metabolically active fraction, referred to as "free testosterone". Only the free testosterone is the biologically active component and affects the sexual function. The relevance of SHBG testing in the process of investigating ED is given below:

- *While evaluating a person's testosterone levels, his SHBG, total testosterone and free testosterone should be determined. This allows clinician to know how much testosterone is being produced and how much free testosterone is bio-available to affect sexual function.*

- *Whenever the total testosterone measurement is not consistent with clinical signs and symptoms, while the patient definitely has signs and symptoms of increased or decreased testosterone, SHBG value can help to determine the value of bioavailable 'free testosterone'.*

- *Measurement of free testosterone is imperative in the diagnosis of many diseases, most significantly disorders of androgen deficiency in men i.e. hypogonadism.*

- *The level of SHBG in our blood changes because of factors such as obesity, hyperthyroidism and liver disease. When our SHBG levels are low, our body has more unbound free testosterone available for use. When our SHBG levels are high, our body has lesser testosterone at its disposal.*

9. **Prostate Specific Antigen (PSA):** This is a blood test. It is a screening test to assess prostate health. PSA is a protein produced by normal prostate gland. It is mainly produced to enable ejaculation, where it helps to liquefy semen and allow sperms to swim freely, thus playing an important role in fertility. The maximum amounts of PSA are found in the semen; some PSA escape the prostate and can be detected in the blood. The relevance of PSA testing in the process of investigating ED is given below:

- *In cases of ED due to low testosterone (hypogonadism), before prescribing testosterone supplements to the patient, it is very important to know the status of the prostate gland.*

- *The PSA is found raised in wide range of conditions besides prostate cancer, such as benign prostatic hyperplasia (BPH), inflammation or infection of the prostate gland (prostatitis), urinary tract infection (UTI), following catheterization or cystoscopy and even digital rectal examination. All these conditions carry the potential to adversely affect erectile function.*

10. **Follicular Stimulating Hormone (FSH):** This test measures the level of Follicle Stimulating Hormone (FSH) in our blood. FSH is produced by our pituitary gland and plays an important role in sexual development and functioning in men as well as in women. The relevance of FSH testing in the process of investigating ED is given below:

- *Low as well as high levels of FSH can cause a variety of problems, including infertility (the inability to get pregnant), low sex drive in men, and early or delayed than expected puberty in growing children.*

- *FSH testing is crucial and fundamental during the evaluation of fertility issues and the health of your reproductive glands (ovaries or testicles) in men as well as women. In men, FSH stimulates as well as controls 'spermatogenesis' i.e. the production of sperms.*

- *FSH is often tested to assess 'pituitary gland functioning' or hypothalamic disorder. The Pituitary gland plays the most important role in the production of 'all' the hormones related to sexual and reproductive functions. Thus, both men and women may need FSH testing if they have symptoms of a pituitary disorder such as weakness, fatigue, weight loss and decreased appetite.*

11. **Luteinizing Hormone (LH):** This test measures the level of Luteinizing Hormone (LH) in our blood. FSH and LH both work in tandem with each other like partners, complementing each other, while doing their own independent jobs. Both are produced by our pituitary gland and play an independent and equally important role in sexual development and reproductive functioning in men as well as in women. The relevance of LH testing in the process of investigating ED is given below:

    - *Low levels of LH in adult males leads to low testosterone levels, causing symptoms such as lack of sexual interest, ED and fatigue.*

    - *High levels of LH indicate primary testicular failure.*

    - *LH is often tested along with FSH to assess 'pituitary gland functioning'. In certain cases when the patient is given the Gonadotropin Releasing Hormone (GnRH) shot and the LH levels either go down or remain the same, it is diagnostic of pituitary disease.*

12. **Serum Prolactin (PRL):** This test measures the level of Prolactin Hormone (PRL) in our blood. Prolactin is produced by our pituitary gland. In females Prolactin causes the breasts to grow and produce milk during pregnancy and after childbirth. The specific function of prolactin in men is not well-understood. However,

prolactin levels have been used to measure sexual satisfaction in men as well as in women. The relevance of Prolactin testing in the process of investigating ED is given below:

- *In men, raised prolactin level can cause decreased libido and/or erectile dysfunction.*

- *High concentration of prolactin in blood interferes with the function of the testicles, the production of testosterone, and sperm production. Low testosterone causes decreased energy, sex drive, muscle mass and strength.*

- *Prolactin is tested to detect and monitor a pituitary tumour that produces prolactin (prolactinoma). Presence of prolactinoma is invariably associated with low sex drive and ED.*

13. **Thyroid Function Tests (T3, T4, TSH):** These are blood tests used to assess how well our thyroid gland is working. The tests include the T3, T4, and TSH. Thyroid hormones are responsible for helping to regulate many of the body's processes, such as metabolism, energy generation, and mood. The relevance of Thyroid Function Tests in the process of investigating ED is given below:

- *Hypothyroidism (underactive thyroid) and Hyperthyroidism (overactive thyroid) are the two thyroid conditions. Both are known for affecting a man's ability to achieve erections. It is found more common in men with hypothyroidism as compared to men with hyperthyroidism.*

- *An effective treatment for both these conditions is available and can significantly correct erection problems.*

14. **Routine Urine test (Urinalysis):** A urinalysis is a test of our urine. It is used to detect, monitor and manage a wide range of disorders, such as urinary tract infections (UTIs), kidney diseases, liver diseases and diabetes. As all these conditions are known to affect erectile function, a urinalysis is always included in the battery of tests done to evaluate ED.

15. **Semen analysis (Seminogram):** A semen analysis is done as part of infertility testing to help evaluate male fertility, whether for those seeking pregnancy or verifying the success of vasectomy. A patient's ability to procure semen sample through masturbation also confirms the patient's ability to get aroused and ejaculate semen, two important aspects of sexual functioning.

<u>When specialized tests are required</u>

In most cases, the history, physical examination, and blood testing allow the physician to identify possible causes of an erectile dysfunction, but in some cases, a more advanced evaluation may be required.

1. **Nocturnal Penile Tumescence (NPT) studies**
2. **Rigi Scan**
3. **Penile Doppler Ultrasonography**
4. **Cavernosography with/without Cavernosometry**
5. **Penile Arteriography**

1. **Nocturnal Penile Tumescence (NPT) studies:** During the treatment if the clinician suspects that the patient has a psychogenic basis for his ED, he may order Nocturnal Penile Tumescence (NPT) studies to confirm this provisional diagnosis. The NPT test involves wearing a specialized device around the penis at night while sleeping. The device records

whether the patient gets erections during his sleep. To get erections during sleep is both common and normal. If NPT studies show that the patient had erections during sleep, it would suggest that his ED is psychogenic in nature. This confirmation can then help the clinician to plan the appropriate treatment strategy. However, NPT studies have its limitations as nocturnal erections may not be the same as sexually induced erections.

2. **The RigiScan:** It was developed as a convenient home device to assess the quality and the quantity of nocturnal erections. It can help to distinguish functional from inadequate erections as well as in distinguishing psychogenic from organic ED. RigiScan records continuous measurements of penile rigidity and tumescence.

More on RigiScan

The RigiScan device consists of a portable battery-operated unit that is strapped around the thigh. It has two loops that are connected to a direct-current torque motor. One loop is placed around the base of the penis and the other is placed just below the glans penis. Every 30 seconds the loops tighten and the penile circumference is measured to estimate tumescence. Fifteen seconds later, a second measurement is taken without actively tightening of the loop. If tumescence gauged by the length of the loop increases by 10 mm or more, than from the initial measurements, rigidity measurements are taken on record. In this manner rigidity measurements are recorded every half a minute by slightly tightening the loops.

The rigidity is mentioned as a percentage, with 100% equating the rigidity of a standard firm noncompressible rubber dummy. The information recorded in the device is then downloaded into a microprocessor, and then analyzed, displayed, and printed in the form of a report. The RigiScan measures only redial rigidity across the girth of the penis. It does not measure axial rigidity across the length of the penis. Axial rigidity is equally important as it tests the ability of the penis to stay straight in spite of pressure against the tip of a penis during penetration.

3. **Penile Doppler ultrasonography:** This is a high-performing, minimally-invasive imaging technique that allows the delineation of the normal anatomy and macroscopic pathological changes in real time. Furthermore, functional changes in the penile blood flow, as seen in ED can also be evaluated by using color Doppler ultrasonography.

This test helps to evaluate the penile vasculature and have a preliminary assessment of the arterial and venous function in the penis.

More on Penile Doppler Ultrasonography

In this study, the patient is injected with a medication that causes smooth muscle relaxation and increases penile blood flow. For the injection, there are options available, such as Alprostadil (Caverject) 10mg or Trimix/Triple P (Prostaglandin E1, Papaverine, and Phentolamine). After the injection, a sonologist performs sequential blood flow studies. The rate at which blood is flowing through the cavernosal artery on each side of the penis (the peak systolic velocity) can be measured. A peak systolic velocity over 25 to 30 ml/sec is regarded as normal. The Doppler ultrasound also helps to measure the diameter of the cavernosal arteries. In addition, the functioning of the penile veins can also be evaluated by measuring the end-diastolic velocity i.e. venous resistance. This procedure carries a small risk of priapism and penile pain related to the injection. If the Doppler ultrasound study demonstrates an abnormality of the arteries or veins, a corrective surgery then can be advised.

4. **Cavernosography:** It is a specialized test for ED. It is used in cases where the cause of ED is suspected to be a venous leak (veno-occlusive dysfunction) and the surgical repair (venous ligation procedures) is being considered. This test is performed by injecting either with 10 micrograms of Alprostadil or a similar dose of Trimix/Triple 3 into Corpora Cavernosa by using a butterfly needle. The needle is placed into the corpora. A contrast material is infused through the needle, and x-ray images are obtained periodically during the infusion. This facilitates viewing of the exact sites of venous leakage.

5. **Cavernosometry:** This test is similar to Cavernosography and is often done along with Cavernosography. It is performed in the similar manner by first injecting either 10 mg of Alprostadil or an equivalent amount of Trimix/Triple P and then placing a small butterfly needle into corpora cavernosa on either side of the penis, one for saline infusion and the other one for pressure monitoring. The speed of infusion that is necessary to initiate and then maintain an erection is noted down. A failure to produce a satisfactory rigid erection or to increase the intracavernous pressure to 90 mmHg or higher, despite an increase in the speed of infusion to 300ml/minute is diagnostic of a veno-occlusive dysfunction i.e. venous leak. Likewise, a quick decrease in pressure in the corpora cavernosa once

the infusion is stopped is also indicative of a venous leak. This test is not advised routinely in all men with a provisional diagnosis of venous leak; rather, it is performed in select men who wish to pursue possible surgical repair.

6. **Penile Arteriography:** This test is performed to identify and localize arterial disease. It is performed with an injected agent that stimulates blood flow, such as Alprostadil or Trimix/Triple P. Invariably a **Penile Doppler ultrasonography** is done before the penile arteriography to identify arterial inflow problems. Only those select individuals who are open to a possible 'penile bypass surgery' as a treatment option are advised penile arteriography. The ideal candidate for penile arteriography followed by penile bypass surgery is a healthy young man with a prior history of trauma leading to ED.

   Penile arteriography is a gold standard investigation but one of the most challenging vascular studies to perform. Thus, it should be performed only by an expert and experienced interventional radiologist or a cardiologist.

   The procedure is performed under local anesthesia. A dose of 10 mg of Alprostadil or an equivalent amount of Trimix/Triple P is injected into the side of the penis to maximize blood flow to the penis. A needle is then passed into the femoral artery in the groin area, and a small catheter is passed through the needle. Under radiological monitoring the catheter is then advanced until it is in a correct location for injection of the contrast agent. Contrast is then injected for the x-ray visualization of the arteries to identify and locate arterial inflow problems.

Chapter 5
Treating Erectile Dysfunction

Overview of Treatment options in Erectile Dysfunction

For a man who is experiencing Erectile Dysfunction (ED), the first and the foremost thing to do is to approach a qualified doctor with authentic credentials and good standing in the field.

The good news is that there is a wide range of treatment options that are available for Erectile Dysfunction (ED), and most people with ED will find a solution that works for them.

Most types of sexual dysfunction can be addressed by treating the underlying physical or psychological problems.

The treatment for erectile dysfunction in particular often begins with taking good care of your heart and vascular health. *"What is good for your heart is good for your penis (erection)"* - is my quote that had gone viral in the media way back in 2014. A treating doctor needs to begin with pointing out 'risk factors' that need to be modified, changed, eliminated and/or improved to enhance cardio-vascular health.

Research has shown that sedentary lifestyle (inactivity) and obesity (excess weight) are the two risk factors for many different conditions that may lead to Erectile Dysfunction. Smoking also increases the risk of developing atherosclerosis which can further contribute to ED. Patients may be thus asked to change certain food habits, quit smoking, exercise regularly, stop using alcohol and some other recreational drugs and change certain medications. Often offering alternative medication is easily possible and can bring about significant improvement in the quality of an erection.

A proper study published in *The Journal of Sexual Medicine* in May 2014 found that some men can actually 'reverse' ED with healthy lifestyle choices, such as regular exercise, losing weight, following a proper diet plan and good sleep. Some Australian researchers have also demonstrated that even if medication may be required, it is more effective if one implements certain healthy lifestyle changes.

The treating doctor may also offer some relevant 'sex education' and suggest addressing emotional and psychological problems, which could stem from relationship conflicts, work pressure, life's stressors, anxiety or depression due to unresolved issues and past trauma.

Ahead of addressing the above mentioned primary and immediate concerns, sincere efforts are then taken by a treating doctor nevertheless to get the 'definitive diagnosis' i.e. exact cause/s of ED. This makes it rather smooth and straight forward for the diagnosis and to begin the specific treatment to treat the cause.

The success rates of treatment also depend on the causes and the degree of erectile dysfunction. Knowing the origin of the problem guides the treating doctor to determine the likelihood of success of a chosen line of treatment and to avoid falsely elevated unrealistic expectations.

It helps significantly to involve the patient's spouse/partner in the evaluation and the treatment process of ED. In realistic terms, therapist's intervention is less likely to succeed if the partner does not show interest in resuming sexual relations.

For example, if the partner has reached menopause and is suffering from Atrophic Vaginitis (a common form of female sexual dysfunction in postmenopausal women), she may find peno-vaginal intercourse uncomfortable and thus may not be inclined to be supportive in the treatment of ED.

Atrophic vaginitis is common among post-menopausal women. It occurs due to lower estrogen levels that make vaginal mucosa to become thin, dry and prone to irritation. Involving both the partners in treatment can open up an opportunity to address both problems - ED as well as Atrophic vaginitis. The discomfort from Atrophic Vaginitis can be helped by using commonly available topical estrogen cream which helps restore the vaginal mucosa. In addition, the concurrent use of an appropriate artificial lubricant during peno-vaginal intercourse can further minimize the discomfort during intercourse. Topical estrogen cream can however be advised only after careful individual assessment of risks and benefits of using it.

In most of the cases of ED, once the possible causes are identified and evaluated, the doctor educates the patient about the lifestyle changes he needs to bring about and also the possible treatment options. This type of a goal-oriented approach focuses on the doctor-patient discussing the possible causes of the problem and then making a decision about the various treatment options. Younger men with no identifiable medical conditions or risk factors are advised to undergo further evaluation as they make better candidates for penile vascular surgery.

In those cases where there is a significant psychogenic component to the erectile dysfunction, then it can be best dealt with counselling/psychotherapy, supportive therapy and relevant sex education. If ED is due to a situational cause, the treatment will be predominantly 'sex counselling' and 'supportive therapy'. If the cause is organic, then appropriate medical or surgical measures will have to be undertaken. Even in those men where organic problem is identified and treated, realistically, in most men there is always some psychological overlay. Treating the organic cause of ED also helps to resolve psychogenic problems arising out of erectile dysfunction. However, if there are significant psychological stressors, then counselling alongside the medical line of treatment can be more helpful than medical line of treatment alone.

Treatment options for ED

In many cultures and societies, even in todays day and age, problems related to sexual functions are not discussed openly. This has made research into the pathophysiology and treatment of ED develop slower than many other branches of medicine. This resulted into massive exploitation, blatant quackery, unrealistic claims and fake treatment options for ED. However, with the advent of oral therapy and vast media-driven social awareness about Sildenafil Citrate (Viagra) as the first ever effective oral treatment available for ED, there is now a heightened interest, openness and a willingness to come out in the open to discuss ED. Before the advent of oral therapy, only about 5-10% of men with ED would seek help, however with the advent of oral therapy, around 15-20% men with ED are now seeking help.

Erectile dysfunction is not a disease in and of itself, rather, it is a symptom or a manifestation of an underlying disease process. Thus, it is imperative to take all the efforts to search for these underlying disease processes that cause ED during the history taking, while investigating and conducting the physical examination, because many of these diseases such as Diabetes Mellitus, Dyslipidemia, and Coronary Artery Disease (CAD) are associated with significant morbidity and possible mortality.

Furthermore, ED is also known to have a significant impact on the quality of life, self-esteem, prevalence of depression, and the quality of relationship with the partner. Thus, the treatment of ED and the underlying causative disease processes can have a major impact on the overall well-being of the man and even his partner.

The choice of the appropriate treatment for each patient depends on multiple factors such as medical, cultural, ethnic, religious, personal and financial. Each treatment option has its own advantages and disadvantages that makes it either more or less suitable for individual patients.

Potentially modifiable risk factors comprise:

- **Lifestyle changes**: Weight loss, quit smoking and other recreational drugs, reduce alcohol consumption, diet modification to manage diabetes and control cholesterol and triglyceride levels, better time management and even changing of the bicycle seat.

- **Improving psychosocial factors**: Resolving conflicts with the partner, seek couple counselling, manage stress, treatment for anxiety or depression etc.

- **Sex education**: Learning about sexual needs of self and the other, understanding the sexual response cycle, knowledge about age-related changes in the sexual function and learn and understand about the cause of the problem from expert.

- **Reviewing iatrogenic causes of ED**: ED may be the result of certain medications, diagnostic procedures and surgical interventions.

Not all men with erectile dysfunction will be able to restore their erectile function completely and permanently. If the cause of your ED is suspected to be psychogenic (originating from the mind), then counselling and psychotherapy would be a first-line therapy. It is necessary to recognize that psychosocial factors are important in all types of ED, and psychosexual counselling can be of great benefit to the couple with organic ED as well as to those with psychogenic ED.

Currently available therapies for the treatment of organic ED:

- **Oral therapy**: A patient is given oral preparations to manage either the underlying organic cause of ED or then directly treat the symptom of ED. Other oral preparations such as Apomorphine SL, Trazodone and Yohimbine are also offered by some therapists in some countries, however these are not recommended as first-line therapies for ED.

- **Injection therapy**: Papaverine, Alprostadil (Prostaglandin E1), Triple P (phentolamine, prostaglandin, and papaverine), and Bimix (papaverine and phentolamine) are used in injection therapy for intrapenile injections to achieve an erection.

- **Mechanical therapy**: The Vacuum device is the most commonly advised mechanical therapy for ED.

- **Surgical therapy**: A smaller percentage of men with identifiable vascular cause and no other underlying medical condition may be good candidates for surgical options. Venous ligation surgery (Venous leak corrective surgery), Penile bypass surgery (Arterial revascularization surgery), Penile prosthesis are the available surgical options.

It is important for the treating doctor to discuss all treatment options with the patient and to inform and educate the patient about all the pros and cons of each.

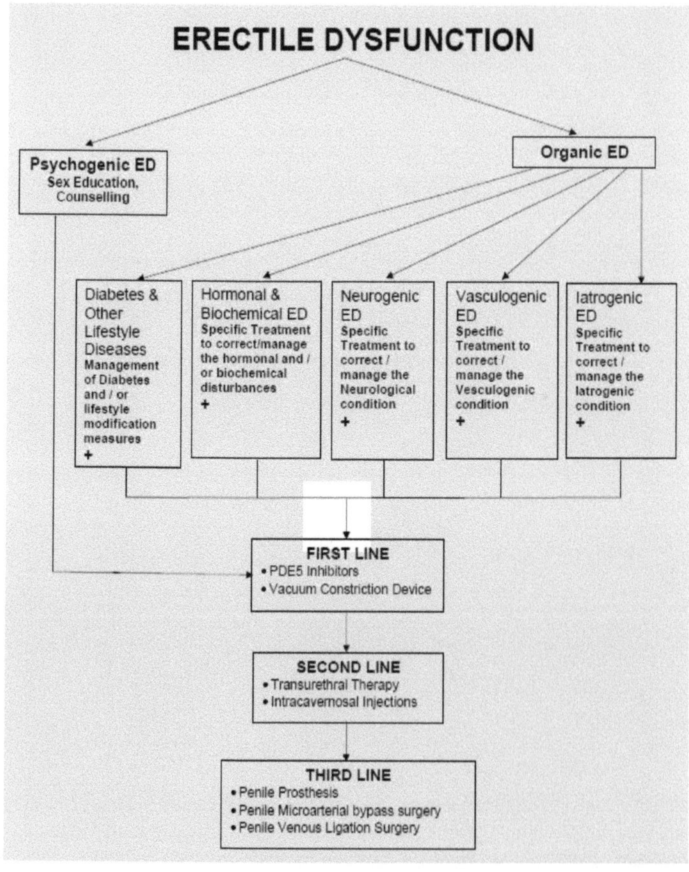

Chapter 6
Oral Therapy for Erectile Dysfunction

*Pharmacological Innovations in
Phosphodiesterase Type 5 Inhibition*

History of Oral PDE5 Inhibitors

In the mid-1980s, the numerous physiological effects of Nitric Oxide (NO) had dramatic implications for a number of diseases. The PDE enzyme is ubiquitous in the body. The PDE5 enzyme is widespread but is more prevalent in penile tissue. Since then, a number of selective PDE inhibitors have been approved to treat a variety of disorders ranging from ED to pulmonary hypertension.

Sildenafil was first studied in clinical trials in 1991 for coronary heart disease. However, the drug surprisingly was found to have favourable effects on penile erections. By 1998, Sildenafil, popularly known by the brand name Viagra was FDA-approved as the first oral treatment for ED. It is the most commonly used first-line therapy for the treatment of ED in men who have no contraindication for its use.

As realization of the market potential for oral PDE5 inhibitors emerged, pharmaceutical companies were now set out to bring new variations and improvements. Different potencies, onsets of action and durations of action played into the producing alternative PDE5 inhibitors. Tadalafil and Vardenafil came in 2003, and Avanafil followed in 2012 for treatment of ED.

How Sildenafil helps

To understand how Sildenafil helps, it is important to first quickly review the processes involved in the normal erection. When sexually aroused or stimulated, our brain sends out messages that lead to an increase in the release of Nitric Oxide from the pelvic nerves. This nitric oxide then further stimulates the production of a chemical called cGMP, which in turn directs the cavernosal smooth muscle and the cavernosal arteries to relax and dilate, thus causing increased blood flow to the penis. Subsequently cGMP is broken down by the enzyme Phosphodiesterase type 5 (PDE5).

Sildenafil stops PDE5. This makes cGMP to stay available for a longer time to continue to provide stimulation to the cavernosal smooth muscle and arteries, thereby sustaining adequate blood flow into the penis. Sildenafil cannot bring about an artificial erection in a flaccid penis. Critical to the success of Sildenafil is the need for an independent sexual arousal and/or sexual stimulation, so that the brain will stimulate the release of nitric oxide. In other words, Sildenafil only helps to 'sustain' the existing erection for a longer duration. It is not of much use in those men who have difficulty in 'getting' an erection. It helps only those who get an erection 'on their own' but cannot sustain it long enough to perform satisfactory sexual intercourse.

Who can take Sildenafil?

Most men below the age of 65 can safely take Sildenafil. The safety of Sildenafil has not been officially studied and documented adequately and systematically for men above sixty-five years of age, though individual data and observations of many practicing doctors and patients have shown good tolerance for Sildenafil in men above 65.

There are definite contraindications to the use of Sildenafil, and if these are not adhered to, serious life-threatening side effect problems can arise.

Effectiveness of Sildenafil against the Cause of ED

Cause	Success Rate	Source and Study
General Population	70 %	*New England Journal of Medicine 1998; 338:1397-1404*
Psychogenic	73 – 89 %	*International Journal of Impotence Research 1998; 10:53, 254a*
Hypertension	70 %	*New England Journal of Medicine 1998; 338:1397-1404*
Diabetes Mellitus	50 – 65 %	*JAMA 1999; 281:421-426*
Spinal Cord Injury	57 – 93 %	*European Urology 2000; 38:134-193*
Myelomeningocele (Spina Bifida)	80 %	*Journal of Urology 2000; 163 (3, part 2): 958-961*
Multiple Sclerosis	90 %	*Urologic Clinics of North America 2001; 32:289-308*
Radiation for Prostate Cancer	70 – 80 %	*Journal of Clinical Oncology 1999; 17:3444-3449*

Contraindications to the use of Sildenafil include:

- Organic **Nitrates** (which are a form of nitric acid that causes dilatation of the coronary arteries of the heart), and **Nitrites** should not be used for angina pectoris for at least 24 hours after Sildenafil is ingested. The reason for this is that when combined, the combination of Sildenafil and Nitrates may lower blood pressure to a dangerous level, making it a life-threatening combination. Thus, concurrent use of preparations that contain organic Nitrates or Nitrites such as sublingual nitroglycerin or nitroglycerin patch, amyl nitrates, long-acting nitrates etc with Sildenafil is to be strictly avoided
- Recent episode of Myocardial Infarction
- Congestive Cardiac Failure (inability of the heart to effectively pump blood, leading to swelling and fluid collection in the lungs) with a borderline low blood volume
- Severe Cardiac Arrhythmias (irregular heartbeats)
- A medical condition that can make a man predisposed to Priapism, such as sickle cell disease and trait, leukemia and multiple myeloma
- Retinitis Pigmentosa (a congenital eye condition that causes blindness).

If the patient is unsure of his cardiac status or has a strong family history of cardiovascular disease, then he needs to go for further cardiac evaluation before using Sildenafil. A cardiac stress test can be advised to assess the cardiac risks associated with the use of Sildenafil.

An extremely rare vision problem called NAION (Nonarteritic Anterior Ischemic Optic Neuropathy) – was reported by a few men using these drugs.

The condition NAION causes a sudden loss of eyesight as blood flow gets blocked to the optic nerve. People who have a higher chance for NAION include those who:

- Smoke

- Are above 50 years of age

- Have a history of diabetes, high blood pressure, dyslipidemia (high lipid levels) and heart disease

- Have certain preexisting eye problems

Several observational studies were done and published in June 2018. These studies could not find an association between NAION and PDE5 use.

Some more cautions about prescribing Sildenafil

Sildenafil should not be taken more than once in a 24-hour period.

Sildenafil is either not to be given to men over 65 years of age, or given with utmost caution and responsibility on the part of the treating physician.

Several medications increase the level of Sildenafil in plasma, sometimes even higher than in men who are taking a 100 mg of Sildenafil. These drugs include Cimetidine, Clarithromycin, Erythromycin, Itraconazole, Ketoconazole, and the range of protease inhibitors (drugs that strongly inhibit the CYP24A liver enzyme, generally prescribed for HIV/AIDS) such as Ritonavir, Indinavir, Saquinavir and Nelfinavir. Sildenafil can best be avoided with men on these medications or could be started at a dose of 25 mg. Men taking Ritonavir (the most potent of all protease inhibitors), are suggested to take Sildenafil not more than once every 48 hours.

Alcohol and Sildenafil

A very frequently asked question by patients as well as fellow medicos, whether Sildenafil can be taken along with alcoholic drink/s. The answer is YES. Sildenafil can safely be taken with a glass of beer or a wine or a mixed alcoholic drink. Their actions do not interfere with each other.

However, excess alcohol intake can independently have a negative effect on erectile function and thus, one needs to limit one's alcohol intake.

Food and Sildenafil

A *fatty meal* around the time of Sildenafil can cause slow absorption of the drug. This can cause delay its time of onset of action.

Also, *diabetic men* who experience *slow gastric emptying* (food takes longer time to move through their stomach) may need to take the pill a couple of more hours before anticipated intercourse.

How to take Sildenafil tablet?

Once indicated, Sildenafil is always taken on demand, meaning that each time one wishes to have penetrative intercourse, he is required to take a pill.

The pill is to be swallowed ½ hour to 1½ hours prior to anticipated time of the intercourse. However, realistically speaking, it can very well be taken up to 3 to 5 hours before anticipated intercourse.

Sildenafil can be taken in four different doses of 25, 50, 75 and 100 mg. It is best to start with 25 mg. This is found effective in most men. Particularly those men with impaired renal function or a liver disease, and those who are using medications that can increase the concentration of Sildenafil in the blood, it is safer to start with 25 mg. If there is either no response or an inadequate response to 25 mg, then the physician can prescribe a higher dose of 50, 75 and 100 mg as per the requirement.

It is necessary to remember, that Sildenafil merely facilitates your body's response, and thus it definitely requires proactive sexual stimulation for it to work. Without sexual stimulation, physical or mental, Sildenafil would not bring about any erectile response. Thus, either self-pleasuring or a foreplay with a partner, or mental stimulation such as thinking, watching, visualizing or a fantasy of sex are necessary for Sildenafil to be effective and come into action.

Common side effects of Sildenafil

Nasal congestion, flushing and headache are the most common side effects of Sildenafil. These are all vasodilatory effects i.e. dilation of blood vessels. Isolated episodes of temporary hemorrhoidal bleeding and a skin reaction have also been reported with the use of Sildenafil.

Gastroesophageal reflux disease (GERD) can also occur as a result of dilation of the gastroesophageal sphincter.

Visual side effects include change in color vision (green-blue discrimination), due to inhibitory effect of Sildenafil on PDE6 photoreceptors in the eye. Other visual disturbance that have been reported include redness, burning, diplopia (double vision) and even temporary loss of vision. The visual side effects are always transient and reversible. Long-standing changes in the vision have not been reported. Sildenafil also does not increase intraocular pressure.

During therapeutic use, Sildenafil is also found to produce a non-dose-related drop in blood pressure. While Systolic BP may drop by 8 to 10 mm of Hg, the Diastolic BP may drop by and 5 to 6 mm of Hg. In most cases, this drop may not cause any significant side effects; however, men who are taking three or more antihypertensive medications, this mild drop in BP may be significant.

Tachyphylaxis and Sildenafil

Tachyphylaxis means diminishing response to successive doses of a drug, rendering it less and less effective. In simple terms, the medication works well initially but after using it for a short period of time, the same dose of medication is not effective anymore.

There are several reports of tachyphylaxis to Sildenafil. It is still rather unclear whether or not the reported incidents are truly cases of tachyphylaxis, or a result of progression of the erectile dysfunction.

Tadalafil

Tadalafil is another PDE5 inhibitor that is effective and found effective in the treatment of erectile dysfunction. Both Tadalafil and Sildenafil have proven to have similar success rates in clinical trials i.e. effective in over 80% of those that use either drug. However, a clinical trial done in Italy showed that 73% of men preferred Tadalafil over Sildenafil.

Effect of Tadalafil lasts longer than Sildenafil. Sildenafil has a duration of action for up to 4 hours, whereas effect of Tadalafil can last for up to 36 hours. Tadalafil works quicker than Sildenafil by around 10-20 minutes. Sildenafil works around 30-60 minutes after it has been ingested, whereas Tadalafil works around 20-30 minutes after it has been consumed. Both Sildenafil and Tadalafil work best on an empty stomach.

Tadalafil 2.5 mg and 5 mg can be taken every day, and is best suited for those that have more than two sexual intercourses per week.

Both Tadalafil and Sildenafil have a similar side-effect profile, but the side-effects of Tadalafil may last longer, due to its longer window of action. However, Sildenafil has a longer list of side-effects that don't appear to be as common in Tadalafil. A common side-effect of both, includes headache. You may also encounter facial flushing. Nasal congestion is another common side-effect of Tadalafil as well as Sildenafil.

Property	Sildenafil	Vardenafil	Tadalafil	Avanafil
Year of Authorization	*1998*	*2003*	*2003*	*2013*
Onset of action	*30-60 minutes*	*30-60 minutes*	*60-120 minutes*	*15-30 minutes*
Duration of action	*4-12 hours*	*4-10 hours*	*Up to 36 hours*	*Up to 6 hours*
Marketed dosages	*25, 50, 100 mg*	*5, 10, 20 mg*	*2.5, 5, 10, 20 mg*	*50, 100, 200 mg*
Effect of food intake	*High-fat meals decreases efficacy*	*High-fat meals decreases efficacy*	*Nil*	*Nil*

Chapter 7
Vacuum Constriction Device

Mechanical Therapy for Erectile Dysfunction

A Vacuum Constriction Device (VCD) is an external pump with a band (constriction ring) on it that a man with erectile dysfunction can use to get and maintain his erection.

The function of the VCD is based on two principles:

1. Vacuum, or negative pressure, is created to pull blood into the penis.
2. A constriction device (band) is used at the base of the penis to prevent venous drainage and thus prolong the erection.

The VCD consists of an acrylic cylinder with a pump that can be directly attached to the end of the penis. The cylinder is wide enough and long enough to accommodate the erect penis.

A band is placed on the cylinder at the other end, which is applied to the body. The cylinder and pump create a vacuum and helps the penis to get erect; and a band attached to the pump helps to maintain the erection. The pump is either battery or hand operated. It is a non-invasive, reliable, safe and reversible, method of achieving an erection. The very concept of producing an erection by creating a negative pressure to 'pull blood into the penis' was first described way back in 1874. However, it was in 1974 **Osbon** developed the first commercially available vacuum constriction device. Initially the device did not get FDA approval until 1982. However, by 1990 it was one of the most commonly recommended treatments for erectile dysfunction. It is observed that about 50-80% of men are satisfied with the results of VCDs.

How to use a VCD?

- Place the pump over the penis, which can be pumped either by hand or can run on batteries.
- Air is pumped out of the cylinder to create vacuum. The vacuum draws blood into the shaft of the penis and helps it to achieve an erection.
- Once the penis is erect, with the help of a lubricant, the constriction ring (retaining band) is slid down onto the lower end of the penis.
- The pump is then removed after releasing the vacuum.

Intercourse can then be performed with the constriction ring in place to help maintain the erection. The ring can be left on safely for up to 30 minutes to allow for a successful intercourse.

Be sure that the device has a 'quick release' feature, as there have been reports of penile injuries due to devices that did not release its vacuum on-demand or then released it very slowly.

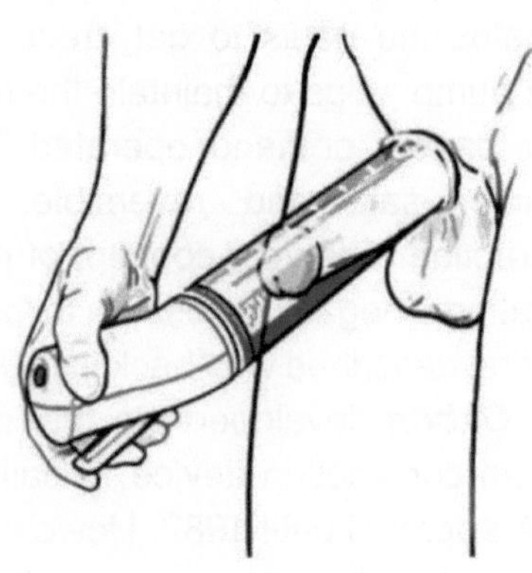

Important points to understand and remember

An erection achieved by the VCD is not the same as an erection achieved naturally. The penis tends to look purplish in color and can be numb and/or cold.

The constriction ring can trap the ejaculate at the time of orgasm. There is also a decrease in the force of ejaculation. This is not harmful and usually may not cause any pain.
The semen dribbles out once the constriction band is removed. However, this does not interfere with the pleasure of an orgasm or climax.

Conditions in which VCD needs extra caution and/or consideration

Vacuum constriction devices should not be used by men who have a significant congenital bleeding disorder.

VCD should also not be used by men with disorders that could predispose them to 'Priapism'. Men with sickle cell anaemia, some forms of leukaemia, and some other blood conditions are prone to develop priapism.

Ischemia of the penis leading to necrosis can occur if the constricting ring is left on for too long. This could particularly be a problem in men with spinal cord injuries, as they do not feel the discomfort related to the constriction ring. If the band is taken off within 30 minutes of application, the risk of penile ischemia is rare.

VCD may be difficult to use in some obese men, due to fatty tissue in their lower abdominal region.

Chapter 8
Intraurethral Alprostadil

Medicated Urethral System for Erections

Intraurethral Alprostadil (MUSE) is an intraurethral medication that was approved by the FDA in June 1998. MUSE stands for Medicated Urethral System for Erections.

Alprostadil (al PROS ta dil) is a synthetic vasodilator, chemically identical to the naturally occurring prostaglandin E(1). Alprostadil stimulates the production of a chemical called cAMP, which, just like cGMP, relaxes blood vessels and muscles in the penis which in turn increases blood flow into the penis, causing an erection.

Alprostadil (MUSE) is an on-demand medication. It needs to be taken each time that you wish to achieve an erection. The success rate has been found ranging from 30 to 64% in various studies. It is available as the single-use pellet (suppository) enclosed in a small applicator.

How to use: The patient is instructed to pass urine before inserting the tip of the applicator into the urethra. Voiding helps lubricate the urethra. Other synthetic topical lubricants such as KY Jelly, petroleum jelly should not be used, as they can hamper the absorption of the alprostadil. Once the applicator is placed into the urethra, the small round button at the end is squeezed to release the suppository into the urethra.

Gently moving the applicator from side to side ensures that the suppository disengages form the applicator and stays within the urethra when the applicator is withdrawn. Once the applicator is removed, gentle massaging of the penis would help the suppository to dissolve in the urethra.

The alprostadil then gets absorbed through the urethral tissue and travels via blood vessels into the corpora cavernosa. Once in the corpora cavernosa, in the next 8 to 20 minutes, the alprostadil causes relaxation of the cavernosal smooth muscle and dilatation of the arteries. This results in penile erection. The duration of the erectile response varies with the dose and could range from 60 to 80 minutes.

In developed countries, intraurethral Alprostadil (MUSE) has found wider acceptance as against intracavernosal injection due to its ease of administration.

There are several different doses of alprostadil (MUSE) available - 125, 250, 500, and 1000 µg. It needs to be refrigerated. It is recommended that the administration of intraurethral alprostadil be initiated at a dose of 500 µg. It has a fast onset of effect and a good safety profile, with no occurrences of fibrosis, priapism, as compared to systemic effects observed with oral treatment with PDE5 inhibitors.

At 500 µg it has a higher efficacy than the 250 µg dose, with minimal differences in adverse events. Intraurethral alprostadil can be administered in all patients irrespective of the cause of ED and could be the first option in patients with ED for whom oral therapy with PDE5 inhibitor is either contraindicated or has failed.

A combination treatment of Alprostadil with PDE5 inhibitor is also emerging as a possible efficient alternative when single oral or intraurethral treatment has failed.

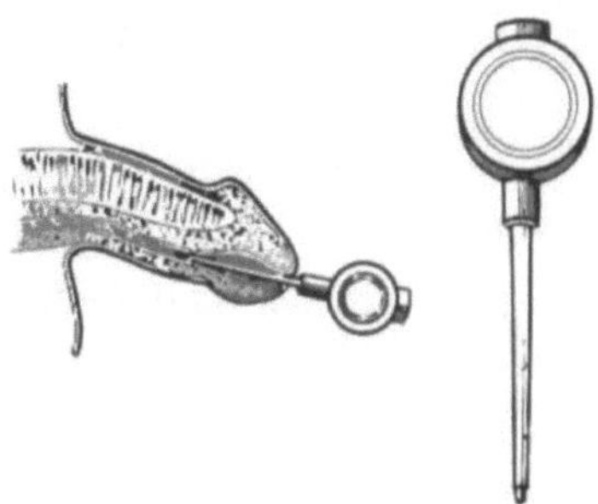

Side effects & Contraindications of Alprostadil (MUSE)

- **Pain and Burning** The most common side effects of Alprostadil is pain and/or burning, found in 30 to 50% users. This may be experienced in the urethra, penis, testes or even the perineum. The intensity of the pain and burning varies, and often depends on the administered dose.

  Men who have undergone radical prostatectomy surgery are likely to have an increased probability of urethral or penile burning and/or pain with Alprostadil and could be warned of this. It is either due to postsurgical hyper-sensitivity of the corpora or due to increased retention of the Alprostadil in the penis as the dorsal vein is often tied off at the time of radical prostatectomy.

- **Urethral bleeding** occurs in 4 to 5% of men.

- **Hypotension** and **Syncopal episodes:** (transient loss of consciousness due to reduced blood flow to the brain) are reported in 1.2 to 4% of men.

- **Dizziness** experiences are seen in 1% of men.

- **Urinary tract infection** is seen in 0.2% of men.

- **Priapism** and **Penile Fibrosis** (scarring) are very rare. Men with sickle cell anemia, polycythemia, thrombocythemia, leukemia or multiple myeloma are at a higher risk for priapism, and can avoid using Alprostadil.

- *About 8-10% of female partners experience vaginal irritation or vaginitis.*

- *Men in whom sexual activity is not advisable, such as those with severe cardiovascular disease, should not use Alprostadil.*

- *It can best be avoided during sex with pregnant partners.*

Chapter 9
Penile Injection Therapy

Intracavernosal Injection Therapy for Erectile Dysfunction

For many years, we have been using medications that improve blood vessel circulation in the penis. They work by relaxing the smooth muscle of the blood vessel walls, causing them to dilate and fill the penis with blood, thus causing erection. Medications such as Sildenafil and Tadalafil (Viagra, Cialis or Levitra) do exactly that, however they may not work for every man dealing with ED.

Penile injection therapy or intracavernosal injection therapy is yet another treatment option for men with ED. Penile injection therapy is the process whereby a small amount of a special chemical is injected directly into the corpora cavernosa of the penis. These chemicals are smooth muscle relaxants and thus help increase blood flow into the penis. It thus helps the man to have an erection and thus perform penetrative intercourse. Since 1983, the Penile Injection Therapy have gained acceptance across the globe. In 1995, the FDA approved Prostaglandin E1 for the treatment of ED.

Having erections regularly keeps erectile tissue in the penis healthy. The tissue in male penis that causes erection (erectile tissue) is composed of smooth muscles (cavernous smooth musculature and the smooth *muscles* of the arteriolar and arterial walls). Going long periods of time without getting an erection is unhealthy for this erectile tissue (smooth muscles) and may slowly cause impairment in its functioning.

Injectable therapies produce a spontaneous erection without the need for any sexual thoughts, feelings or physical stimulation. This is in contrast to oral medications such as Sildenafil (Viagra), which require 'sexual stimulation' to produce an erection. Injectable therapy also overcomes drug absorption issues that can occur with some oral medications.

The thought of putting a needle into your penis may sound intimidating to some people, but about 70% of men are quite satisfied with this therapy.

The three most commonly used medications for injection therapy are:

- **Trimix** – alprostadil (Prostaglandin E1), phentolamine, and papaverine

- **Bimix** – Papaverine HCL, Phentolamine Mesylate

- **Papaverine**

For most men injection therapy begins with Trimix. These ingredients work by relaxing the smooth muscle and opening the blood vessels in the penis, causing an erection.

How Medication Is Injected

First, the medication is drawn into an insulin-type small syringe, with a short, and very fine needle. The volume that you will be injecting is usually 1 cc or less. It does not need to pierce deeply into the penis, just into the corpora on one side, for it to be effective. The syringe used is small also because the volume that is injected is usually 1 cc or less.

The medication is injected along either lateral side of the penis. It is given into the spongy tissue of the penis (corpora cavernosa). It is not necessary to pierce deeply into the penis, just into the corpora on one side, for it to be effective.

Before the patient starts to use penile injection therapy at home, he needs to be test dosed in the doctor's clinic. Out of all of the therapies available for ED, penile injection therapy carries the maximum risk of 'priapism', almost up to 2%.

Priapism occurs in most cases with the very first use of intracavernous injection, during the test dose itself. In case of priapism, the erection can easily be brought back down with just an injection of another medication. Thus, test dosing minimizes your risk of having priapism at an inopportune time. Moreover, your doctor can use the test dosing also as a time for giving you the hands-on training. The patient can practically be shown how to inject and actually perform his first self-injection under the guidance of his doctor. This also helps because the first time he performs the self-injection therapy at home, he can get nervous, and having gone through the experience once in doctor's presence can help him to be confident and relaxed.

After his initial test dose, his doctor decides on a dose that he will take initially at home. If this initial dose is not found adequate, he needs not get discouraged. Most of the doctors would prefer to prescribe a dose that is very small to begin with, and then increase it subsequently as required in order to avoid any possibility of priapism.

When the time comes for self-administration of the injection, one has to first look where he is going to inject. He has to ensure, there are no superficial veins are in that area. After deciding the proper site to inject, the site and the area around it has to be cleaned with an alcohol wipe. The needle is then to be inserted through the skin of the penis, and then the medication is injected into the penis. The needle should be inserted straight into the penis at a 90-degree angle. After injecting and then pulling out the needle and syringe, the injection site has to be pressed firmly either with an alcohol pad or with a gauze using the thumb and index finger to compress the area for about five minutes. For patients who are taking blood thinning medication, one may hold such a compression for about 8-12 minutes.

The medication tends to work better if the patient is standing, as it allows more flow of blood into the penis. A gentle massage of the penis may further increase blood flow to the penis and can allow the medication to take effect faster.

Penile injections are generally to be self-administered at home. Because the injection requires some amount of manual dexterity, it is very important that the patient is methodically taught 'self-injection'. For some men, giving a self-injection may be difficult. They may feel anxious and apprehensive about pushing the needle into their own penis. For such patients an 'auto-injector' is now available. Auto-injector is a spring-loaded device that inserts the needle into the penis very quickly, minimizing physical discomfort and psychological hesitancy. This makes the process of self-injection easier.

Another option is to have the man's spouse/partner trained to perform the self-injection. Also, in situations such as the man is obese and has difficulty seeing his penis, even self-injection with auto-injector may be difficult. In such situations, he may have to take the help of his spouse/partner.

After injecting, erections typically takes about 10–15 minutes to develop, lasting for roughly about 30–60 minutes. This much time is invariably enough for a couple to complete the penetrative intercourse.

The dose required to achieve a satisfactory erection varies greatly with the actual cause of the ED. Younger men with spinal cord injury may only require a very small dose (1 ug) of Alprostadil. While older men with diabetes and vascular disease may require much higher dose such as 40 ug of Alprostadil.

Penile injection therapy is helpful in erectile dysfunction of all causes. As it is not dependent on intact nerves, even patients with a neurologic component to their ED also respond well to injection therapy. It has a success rate ranging from 70 to 94%. Moreover, it also does not interfere with the orgasm and/or ejaculation. However, the long-term success of this therapy requires that the patient be comfortable with the injection therapy.

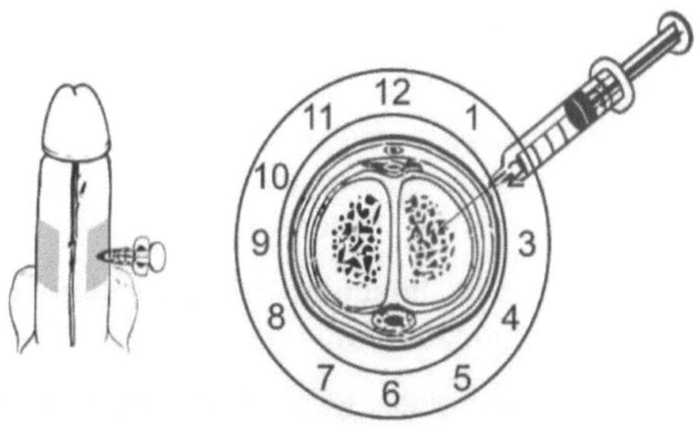

Important points to understand and remember

- Never inject second time once you have injected, even if you feel that you have not injected properly.
- Remember once the medication is constituted i.e., the powder is dissolved in the sterile water, it has to be

refrigerated. The prepared solution loses its efficacy after seven days.

- Make sure that the volume of the medication (dose of medication) that you are injecting is consistent.
- If you are facing any difficulty with self-administering the injections, talk with your doctor. Perhaps getting more instructions or the autoinjector or teaching your spouse/partner would be helpful.
- After injecting the medication, self-stimulation may be necessary to increase the blood flow to your penis.
- Don't inject more often than once in 48 to 72 hours.
- Never reuse needles, and dispose off used needles carefully.
- Always inject on alternate sides during following injections, and not on the same side of penis.
- If your erection lasts more than three hours, call your doctor. Don't wait! Seek medical care at a local emergency room or from your urologist. Waiting will only make it more difficult for your doctor to treat your prolonged erection.
- Remember that your erection may persist even after you have ejaculated and will go down slowly when the medication wears out of your system.

Conditions in which injection therapy needs extra caution and/or consideration

- Men taking an older type of antidepressant, a monoamine oxidase inhibitor such as Isocarboxazid, Tranylcypromine or Phenelzine, should not use injection therapy.
- Men taking blood thinners, such as Warfarin can use injection therapy, but should apply pressure to the injection site for few minutes or so to prevent a bruise.

- Men with Peyronie's disease should be made aware that in the process of injecting, there is local trauma to the tunica albuginea of the penile shaft, which may trigger formation of new plaques.
- Men who are prone to priapism, such as those with sickle cell disease or trait, leukemia and multiple myeloma, these people are at higher risk for priapism if they use injection therapy.
- Penile injections may be ineffective in men who have a vascular disease or blood flow problems.

Low Compliance

In spite of the high efficacy and comparatively low side effects, there is a high discontinuation rate found with injection therapy. It is found that 12-15% of men who are offered injection therapy do not even try it. It is seen that 35-40% men discontinue injection therapy within three months. It is only 20-30% of men who continue with the injection therapy for more than three years.

Reasons for discontinuation

- Problems with ability the to administer the injection
- Fear and pain of needles
- Partner's disapproval or discontent with therapy
- Adverse effects
- Relationship issues with the partner
- No partner
- Return of spontaneous erections

Side Effects

Pain

About 30% of men experience pain with injection therapy. This pain may be at the injection site or a diffused penile pain.

Hematoma

If one does not pay attention closely to where one is injecting, it is possible to injure a superficial vein in the penis, causing hematoma. If this occurs, putting firm pressure on the injection site can stop and prevent further bleeding. Men taking blood thinners need to be extra cautious when injecting and should always apply firm pressure at the injection site after injecting. If there is a significant penile swelling due to hematoma, one should see a urologist.

Priapism

The possibility of priapism with injection therapy is about 2% and most of these cases occur during the first test dose. Trimix carries a slightly higher risk of priapism than Alprostadil. Never inject again after you have injected once, no matter how little you think you injected with the first injection.

Penile Fibrosis

Injection therapy carries a risk of developing 'scar tissue' within the corpora, and this risk is higher with Trimix than with Alprostadil. Over time, this may increase the need to use a higher dose to achieve an adequate erection.

Plaque Formation

One of the concerns with injection therapy is that each time you insert a needle in the tunica albuginea to enter the corpora, it causes minor trauma. This trauma can cause 'plaque' formation, as we see in Peyronie's disease. In view of this potential risk, one should not use injection therapy more frequently than once in 48 hours and should also inject on alternate sides. This helps to evenly distribute the trauma to tunica albuginea and keep the penis from curving to one side.

Occasionally, penile injections can cause dizziness, fainting and low blood pressure.

Chapter 10
Surgical Treatment for ED

When Uro-Surgeon needs to take over

Penile Prosthesis

A Penile prosthesis is an artificial device. It is placed in the penis and allows a man to have an artificial erection. The development and use of penile prosthesis began almost fifty years ago in the 1970s. Since then, modifications and revisions in the prosthesis have steadily improved the satisfaction rate and the mechanical durability of the device.

The first prosthesis developed was a 'rigid' prosthesis. A rigid cylinder was surgically placed into each of the corpora cavernosa. Each cylinder had a fixed girth and length and would remain erect all the times.

The next type of prosthesis that was developed was a 'semirigid' one. The cylinder of the semirigid prosthesis had a flexible metal coil in the center surrounded by silicone. This prosthesis also had a fixed girth and length. However, unlike the rigid prosthesis, it could be bent downwards.

Then came the 'inflatable' prostheses. These are the most commonly used prostheses. They vary from self-contained inflatable protheses to multipart inflatable prostheses. American Medical Systems makes an inflatable prosthesis that has two cylinders. These cylinders have a pump at their tips. When placed into the corpora of the penis, the pump lies in the glans. Gentle squeezing of the glans activates the pump, which then transfers fluid from one compartment of the cylinder to another. This transferring of the fluid causes an erection.

To deflate this prosthesis, the penis is to be bent over one's hand with gentle pressure on the corpora. This manoeuvre drains the fluid back into the other compartment of the cylinder.

Even though this prosthesis is easy to use, the main drawback is that it provides limited girth.

The more commonly used inflatable prostheses are the multipart inflatable prostheses. They are of two types:

1. The two-piece unit, is composed of two cylinders and a combined pump. The reservoir is placed in the scrotum.
2. The three-piece unit, is composed of the two cylinders, a scrotal pump, and a separate reservoir that is placed in the pelvis.

The advantage of the three-piece unit is that it allows the larger amount of fluid transfer, given the larger reservoir size. Moreover, when placed, the device and its tubing are completely concealed. This helps the person to void in any washroom without being noticed.

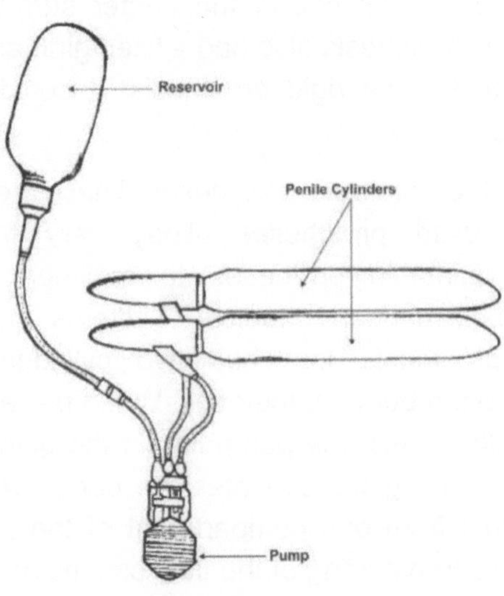

Who is a candidate for a penile prosthesis?

A penile prosthesis is not the first-line therapy for erectile dysfunction. It is chosen in men with organic erectile dysfunction when all other treatment options have either not worked or are contra-indicated. Once the prosthesis is implanted, one cannot go back. If it is removed due to infection, malfunction, or dissatisfaction, all other treatment options are unlikely to work. Thus, it is better to try all other available therapies and determine whether they are successful and satisfactory before implanting a penile prosthesis.

Indications for a penile prosthesis include:

- A patient's dissatisfaction and/or reluctance to consider, failure to respond to, or inability to continue with other forms of treatment, such as oral therapy, injection therapy, MUSE and the vacuum device
- Penile Fibrosis after prolonged use of injection therapy
- Post-priapism ED
- Peyronie's disease causing ED.
- Neurogenic bladder requiring condom catheter for urinary drainage
- Penile amputations in men, who have undergone surgical creation of a neophallus.
- Sex change surgery in women who undergo surgical creation of a neophallus

Penile Microarterial Bypass Surgery (MABS)

Penile Microarterial Bypass Surgery (MABS) also known as Penile revascularization surgery is considered in cases of 'arteriogenic' erectile dysfunction. It is a non-pharmacological, non-device-related, and reconstructive surgical approach for men with ED. This was first described by Dr Vaclav Michal in 1973.

The goal of the penile bypass surgery is to provide an alternate arterial pathway that does not rely on the obstructed artery. This would result in an increased blood flow to the penis so that spontaneous erections can occur.

In view of the technical complexity of the penile bypass surgery, a very small number of men are actually candidates for it.

The ideal candidate is an otherwise healthy man (who has no known medical conditions such as diabetes mellitus, dyslipidemia, hypertension and coronary artery disease) with a distinct arterial occlusive pathology/narrowing in the distal internal pudendal, common penile or proximal cavernosal artery (secondary to focal endothelial injury from blunt pelvic, perineal or penile trauma).

The documented rate of success ranges from 30 to 84%. Careful selection of cases further helps to get optimum long-term results.

The surgery is performed by a trained and experienced uro-surgeon. Some uro-surgeons involve a vascular surgeon for such a procedure. This being a highly specialized procedure, it should be performed by a competent surgeon who has training as well as experience with these types of surgeries. Vascular surgeons perform bypass procedures for blood flow problems throughout the body.

The surgery is performed either under general or spinal anesthesia. Usually two incisions are made, one in the lower abdomen to provide access for the donor artery (the artery that will supply blood into the penis), and another in the opposite groin area to provide access for the recipient artery (the artery to which the donor artery will be connected).

Risk of penile bypass surgery

- Disruption of the anastomosis and consequent bleeding. (The patient is always instructed to avoid intercourse, masturbation, or any heavy activity for six weeks to minimize the risk of injury to the anastomosis).
- Glans hyperemia i.e., increased blood flow to the glans penis. (This occurs in 6 to 14% the of patients).
- Loss of sensation in the penis. (This occurs as a result of nerve trauma during surgery).
- Thrombosis (occlusion) of the bypass graft. (If the blood flow through the graft is not adequate, then thrombosis may occur in the graft).

The risks of penile bypass surgery also include the routine risks of any surgical procedure, bleeding, wound infection, incisional pain and swelling.

Penile Venous Ligation Surgery

Penile Venous Ligation Surgery is another surgical procedure used in chosen cases of erectile dysfunction. It is synonymous with corporoveno-occlusive dysfunction (CVOD). Men whose erectile dysfunction is caused by a 'venous leak' are candidates for this surgery.

In this procedure, the veins that are responsible for the 'venous leak' are first identified and then ligated surgically. Cavernosometry and Cavernosography are the investigations necessary to confirm and establish the presence of a 'venous leak' and to identify the exact site(s) of a venous leak.

Before considering this approach, it is necessary to rule out other arterial diseases that may be occurring along with the venous leak. It is necessary to do an arterial assessment by Colour Doppler sonography before planning this surgery. In addition, there should not be any medical contraindications to the surgery.

Most uro-surgeons do not perform venous ligation procedure. There are very few uro-surgeons who perform this surgery. It is performed either under general or spinal anesthesia. The surgery is performed by taking inguinoscrotal incision that starts in your groin and extends down into the scrotum. It further requires an extensive dissection of the veins, both the superficial as well as deep penile veins. During the surgery, the veins responsible for the venous leak are tied off.

Intraoperative studies are done to delineate the sites of the leakage. At the conclusion of the surgery, they can confirm that a satisfactory erection can be achieved and that there are no residual sites of the venous leak.

The initial reports of short-term results looked promising; however, this effect appears to be lost over time, and the long-term success rate is only about 50%. In men who did not respond over the long–term, new sites of venous leak could be seen on a repeat cavernosography.

Chapter 11
Hypogonadism

Testosterone Deficiency

Hypogonadism occurs when our gonads (sex glands) produce very little or no sex hormones. In men, it is a failure of the testes (gonads) to produce the hormone testosterone, sperms or both. The term 'male hypogonadism', is also often used interchangeably with 'testosterone deficiency'.

In men, testosterone helps to maintain:

- Sex drive
- Bone density
- Fat distribution
- Sperm production
- Facial and body hair
- Red blood cell production
- Muscle strength and muscle mass

Hypogonadism can occur either due to a testicular disorder or the result of a disease process involving the hypothalamus and pituitary gland. It can affect several body functions and can have a negative impact on one's quality of life at various levels. The good news is that most of the cases of hypogonadism respond very well to an appropriate medical line of treatment.

Key features of male hypogonadism:

- Hypogonadism may occur at any age. The consequences depend on when it starts, how long the loss has been occurring, how severe is the deficiency, and whether or not there is a decline in the major functions of the testes

- If hypogonadism occurs before puberty, it affects the progression of puberty. If it occurs after puberty, it causes sexual dysfunction and infertility
- In adult men, signs and symptoms of hypogonadism manifest within a few weeks of the onset of testosterone deficiency
- Hypogonadism may increase the risk of Cardiovascular disease, Type 2 Diabetes, Metabolic syndrome, Alzheimer's disease and premature death in elderly population.

<u>Types of hypogonadism</u>

There are two types of hypogonadism:

1. Primary and
2. Secondary (Central).

Primary hypogonadism

Primary hypogonadism in men means that you don't have enough testosterone in your body due to the malfunctioning of your gonads (testes). It is also known as primary testicular failure as it originates from a problem in the testes. The testes are receiving the signals from your brain to produce testosterone, but they are unable to produce them. This can either be due to a congenital disorder such as undescended testes and Klinefelter's syndrome or due to acquired reasons such as trauma, tumours, mumps infection, radiation therapy or chemotherapy.

Secondary (Central) hypogonadism

In central hypogonadism, the problem lies either in the hypothalamus or in the pituitary gland (parts of the brain that signal the testes to produce testosterone), which are not functioning properly. They are expected to stimulate the testes to start producing testosterone, however they are unable to do that. The hypothalamus produces the Gonadotropin Releasing Hormone (GnRH), which stimulates the pituitary gland to produce the Follicle Stimulating Hormone (FSH) and Luteinizing Hormone (LH). The luteinizing hormone then stimulates the testes to produce testosterone.

Risk factors for hypogonadism

- Stress
- Obesity
- Opioids
- Renal failure
- HIV infection
- Hypertension
- Type 2 Diabetes
- Rapid weight loss
- Glucocorticoid (steroids) intake
- Antipsychotic medication therapy
- Chronic Obstructive Pulmonary Disease (COPD)

Causes of hypogonadism

The causes of primary hypogonadism:

- Trauma to the testes
- Radiation exposure
- Liver and kidney diseases
- Surgery on the sexual organs
- Undescended testes (Cryptorchidism)
- Genetic disorders, such as Klinefelter syndrome
- Severe infections involving testes e.g. Mumps Orchitis
- Autoimmune disorders, such as Addison's disease and hypoparathyroidism

- Hemochromatosis (when our body absorbs excessive iron): Too much iron in the blood can cause testicular failure or pituitary gland dysfunction, affecting testosterone production.

Note on Undescended Testes

Before the birth of a male child, the testes develop inside the lower abdomen of the foetus; and at around birth time they descend into their permanent place in the scrotum. Sometimes, one or both of the testicles may not descend at birth. In most of such cases, the testes descend on their own into the scrotum by the age of 3 to 6 months without any treatment. If not corrected in early childhood, it may lead to malfunction of the testes and decreased testosterone production.

Undescended testes are more often seen in babies who are born early (preterm or premature babies) i.e., before 37 weeks of pregnancy. More commonly just one testis is affected, but in about 10% of the times both testes are undescended.

The causes of secondary (central) hypogonadism:

- Brain surgery
- Cirrhosis of liver
- Pituitary disorders
- Radiation exposure
- Nutritional deficiencies
- Infections, including HIV
- Use of steroids or opioids
- Tumor in or near pituitary gland
- Side effects of certain medications
- Toxins such as alcohol and heavy metals

- Injury to the pituitary gland or hypothalamus

- Genetic disorders e.g. Kallmann syndrome (abnormal hypothalamic development)

- Inflammatory diseases such as tuberculosis, sarcoidosis and histiocytosis can involve the hypothalmus and pituitary gland and can affect the testosterone production, causing hypogonadism.

Note on Andropause

Older men usually have lower levels of testosterone than younger men do. As men age, there is a gradual decrease in the testosterone production. **Andropause** is the term sometimes used to describe decreased testosterone due to the normal ageing process. Starting at approximately 40 years of age, testosterone levels begin to decline at 1.2 - 2% per year. As many as 30% of men older than 75 have a testosterone level that is below normal, according to the American Association of Clinical Endocrinologists.

Symptoms of hypogonadism

Symptoms of hypogonadism i.e., a lack of testosterone can cause a wide range of symptoms in boys/men. The symptoms depend on:

- Age of onset
- Degree of testosterone deficiency
- Duration of testosterone deficiency

1. When the 'Age of onset' for hypogonadism is 'Before Puberty'

If hypogonadism occurs in young adults who have not yet reached puberty, they appear unusually younger than their chronological age.

Their physical development appears stunted as against other children of their age or in comparison with their siblings.

2. When the 'Age of onset' for hypogonadism is 'After the age of Puberty'

- Decreased testicular size
- Enlarged breasts (Gynaecomastia)
- Impaired development of secondary sexual characteristics

3. Symptoms of adult-onset hypogonadism

- Lethargy
- Depression
- Low or no libido
- Erectile Dysfunction
- Low or no sperm count
- Sweating and hot flushes
- Breast enlargement and discomfort
- Decreased muscle mass and strength
- Osteoporosis and reduced bone mineral density
- Lack or Loss of body hair (pubic, axillary, facial)

Tests for hypogonadism

1. Serum Testosterone – Total and Free
2. Sex Hormone Binding Globulin (SHBG)
3. Follicular Stimulating Hormone (FSH)
4. Luteinizing Hormone (LH)
5. Serum Prolactin (PRL)
6. Semen analysis (Seminogram)
7. Complete Blood Count (CBC)
8. Erythrocyte Sedimentation Rate (ESR)
9. Blood Sugar - Fasting and Post-prandial with Urine Sugar
10. Liver Function Tests (Liver Profile)

11. Sonography of Testes and scrotal sacs
12. Testicular biopsy
13. Pituitary imaging – to look for Pituitary gland mass, injury, compression etc
14. Genetic studies – to look for Klinefelter syndrome and Kallmann syndrome (abnormal hypothalamic development) as underlying causes

Note on Genetic conditions that cause Hypogonadism

Klinefelter's Syndrome: This condition results from a congenital chromosomal abnormality of the sex chromosomes - X and Y. Normally men have one X and one Y chromosome. In Klinefelter's syndrome, two X chromosomes (sometime even more) are congenitally present along with one Y chromosome. The Y chromosome carries the genetic material that determines the gender of a child and the associated development. The extra X chromosome affects development of the testes, which consequentially results in the underproduction of testosterone.

Kallmann syndrome: It is a genetic condition that prevents a person from starting or fully completing puberty. To date about 25 different genes have been identified and implicated in causing Kallmann syndrome. It is characterized by abnormal development of the hypothalamus (the part of the brain that controls the secretion of pituitary hormones) causing hypogonadism. Most patients have gonadotropin-releasing hormone (GnRH) deficiency.

This syndrome is also associated with the lack of sense of smell (anosmia) or a reduced sense of smell.

<u>**Treatment of hypogonadism**</u>

Whenever the 'Age of onset' for hypogonadism is 'Before Puberty', it is treated invariably by a qualified pediatric endocrinologist and the treatment is often specific to the individual cause of hypogonadism.

In adult men, the hypogonadism is generally treated with testosterone replacement therapy to bring testosterone levels to normal. Testosterone supplement helps counter the signs and symptoms of male hypogonadism.

It is very necessary to monitor the effectiveness as well as side effects of testosterone replacement treatment several times during the first year of treatment and yearly after that.

Role of Testosterone in the treatment of Erectile Dysfunction

If the patient has erectile dysfunction and his testosterone level is perfectly normal, then giving additional testosterone will have no significant effect on his sexual urge, desire, libido or his quality of erections. If the patient has erectile dysfunction and a low testosterone level, then too giving testosterone supplement alone will most likely not have a significant effect on his erectile function. Therefore, to routinely give testosterone supplement to enhance erectile function is certainly not recommended.

Only in those cases where the cause of erectile dysfunction is secondary to lowered sexual desire and drive (libido), and the testosterone level is concurrently detected to be on a lower side (hypogonadism), then testosterone replacement therapy is considered. However, the benefits of testosterone therapy are always evaluated against potential risks.

Types of Testosterone Replacement Therapy

1. Oral Testosterone preparations were not being used for the treatment of hypogonadism for a long time as they were known for causing serious liver problems. Moreover, they were also not able to keep blood testosterone levels steady.

However, since as recently as March 27, 2019, a new lipophilic testosterone preparation – 'Testosterone Undecanoate' - has become available for oral testosterone replacement treatment with the official approval from United States Food and Drug Administration (FDA). Testosterone undecanoate is a testosterone ester and a prodrug of testosterone. This makes it a natural and bioidentical form of testosterone. Given orally it is absorbed through the intestinal lymphatics, thus by-passing otherwise extensive hepatic first-pass metabolism. This helps to avoid the liver problems that are seen with the other oral testosterone preparations.

2. Transdermal testosterone gels

The need for a transdermal testosterone gel came up mainly to overcome the drawbacks of the other forms of delivery systems. Transdermal gels were launched in the USA in the year 2000. Since then, they have emerged as the most preferred mode of testosterone supplement.

Testosterone gels are available in multiple configurations - 1%; 1.62%; 20 mg/1.25 gm; 25 mg/2.5 gm; 40.5 mg/2.5gm: 50 mg/5 g etc. The generic availability of Testosterone Gel in different configurations is a significant innovation in the testosterone replacement therapy.

The recommended starting dose of testosterone gel is 5 gm/day. This accomplishes a delivery of 5 mg/day i.e., 1%

of testosterone systemically. It is highly recommended that serum testosterone levels should be serially monitored to ensure appropriate dosing. If serum testosterone level remains below the normal range or if the required clinical response is not achieved, the dose may then be increased from 5 gm to 7.5–10 gm.

Better tolerability and dose flexibility makes testosterone gel more acceptable over other modalities of testosterone replacement.

It is advised that testosterone gel be applied in the morning on intact dry skin over the shoulders and upper arms. Application to any other parts of body, such as your penis, scrotum, chest, stomach or armpits is to be absolutely avoided. Patients are instructed to wash their hands thoroughly after application. It is necessary to allow the application site to dry for a couple of minutes and to cover the site with some loose clothing. The patient is instructed to wait for about 4 hours prior to showering. Side effects of gel include skin irritation and the possibility of transferring the gel to another person through contact. The Application site needs to be washed well with soap and water if skin-to-skin contact of these areas is expected with another person.

On application of the gel, serum testosterone levels reach a steady state in the first 24 hours and stay in the normal range for the duration of the application. This pharmacokinetic profile is similar to that of testosterone patch and superior to injectable testosterone esters. Expected rise in PSA (prostate specific antigen) with testosterone therapy is not significantly different with gels. However, the risk of polycythaemia is much lower than injectable testosterone.

3. Testosterone Injections

The most commonly used forms of injectable testosterone replacement therapy, (to treat symptoms of low testosterone in men who have hypogonadism) include 17β-hydroxyl esters of testosterone, administered with oil-based, slow-release vehicles. Commonly used intramuscular-injectable testosterone esters are Testosterone **enanthate**, Testosterone **cypionate**, Testosterone **undecanoate**, and Testosterone **pellet**.

Testosterone **enanthate** and testosterone **pellet** are also used in males with delayed puberty to stimulate puberty.

Testosterone injections work by supplying synthetic testosterone to replace the testosterone that is normally produced naturally in the body. They control symptoms of hypogonadism but do not cure the condition.

Testosterone **enanthate** is one of the **most widely used** intramuscular testosterone esters. At a dose of 200–250 mg, the optimal injection interval is about 2 to 3 weeks; however peak and through values of serum testosterone are often seen above and below the normal range. The suggested dose of testosterone **undecanoate** is 750 mg (3 ml) intramuscularly; followed by 750 mg (3 ml) intramuscularly after 4 weeks, then 750 mg (3 ml) intramuscularly every 10 weeks thereafter.

Other testosterone esters are Testosterone **cypionate** and Testosterone **cyclohexanocarboxylate**. The pharmacokinetics of these testosterone esters are comparable to those of testosterone **enanthate**. Testosterone **cypionate** injection is available in two strengths - 100 mg/ml and 200 mg/ml. Administration of 200 mg of these esters every 2 weeks delivers an adequate form of testosterone replacement.

Testosterone **enanthate**, testosterone **cypionate**, and testosterone **undecanoate** injections are available as a solution to be injected directly into a muscle. Also available as a pellet, it is to be injected under the skin.

Testosterone injection may control the symptoms but will not cure the condition. The doctor may adjust the dose of testosterone depending on the amount of testosterone in the patients' blood during his treatment and his reaction to the medication.

Testosterone propionate is the oldest known testosterone ester, that was discovered in 1936. It was the first testosterone ester that was used in men with hypogonadism, and was the major form of testosterone used until about 1960. It was a short acting oil-based injectable formulation with a terminal half-life of merely 16 to 19 hours. It is not in use anymore and mentioned here only to mark the history.

Some other not-so-prevalent and not-so-popular forms of testosterone therapy in India are given below:

- **Testosterone Patch.** A patch containing testosterone (marketed as Androderm) is applied in the night to patient's torso or thighs. It is found causing severe skin reaction in significant percentage of cases
- **Gum and cheek patch (Buccal rout).** It looks like a tablet, but it sticks to our gum like a patch. It is placed in the vestibule above our top teeth where our gum meets our upper lip in the buccal cavity. This preparation, taken thrice a day, sticks to our gumline and allows testosterone absorption into our bloodstream. It is found causing gum irritation in significant percentage of cases

- **Nasal gel.** This testosterone gel (marketed as Natesto) is pumped into the nostrils - twice in each nostril, thrice in a day. It is more inconvenient than other delivery methods. However, this option minimizes the risk of transferring medication to another person through skin contact
- **Implantable pellets.** Testosterone-containing pellets (marketed as Testopel) are implanted surgically under the skin every three to six months. This rather invasive method of delivery requires an incision

A Note of Caution on Testosterone therapy

A rather tiny percentage of men experience immediate adverse effects of testosterone treatment e.g., acne, breathing disturbances during sleep, swelling and tenderness of breasts, ankles swelling etc. It is also necessary to look for increased red blood cell counts, which can increase the risk of clotting.

Those men who are on a long-term testosterone therapy are at a higher risk of cardiovascular problems such as myocardial infarction and strokes. There is also a concern that testosterone therapy can instigate the growth of prostate cancer cells.

For men with low blood testosterone levels, the benefits of testosterone therapy are always evaluated against potential risks. Thus, for most men, it is always a shared decision with a treating doctor.

Even though testosterone therapy can help to treat low testosterone due to medical conditions, the Food and Drug Administration (FDA) does not advice using it to treat ageing-related natural testosterone decline, as it obviously increases the risk of certain health issues.

Chapter 12
Diabetes and Erectile Dysfunction

How Diabetes Mellitus affects Erectile Ability

Diabetes Mellitus, commonly known as diabetes, is a chronic metabolic disease that causes higher than normal blood sugar levels. It is a condition that weakens the body's ability to process blood glucose, otherwise known as blood sugar.

Blood glucose is our foremost source of energy and comes from the food we eat. All carbohydrate foods we eat are broken down into glucose in the blood. **Insulin**, a hormone produced by the pancreas, acts like a 'key' to open our cells, to allow the sugar (glucose) from the food we eat to enter into the cells in the body to be either stored or used for energy.

Either when the **pancreas** is not able to produce adequate **insulin**, or when the body cannot make good use of the insulin it is producing, the blood glucose starts rising (known as **hyperglycaemia**) beyond normal level. This is called as Diabetes Mellitus. Untreated high blood sugar from diabetes can damage our nerves, blood vessels, kidneys, eyes and various other organs.

There are two predominant types of diabetes mellitus that are related to erectile dysfunction:

Type I Diabetes: It is known as insulin-dependent diabetes or juvenile diabetes. It usually develops in children and teenagers; but people of all ages can develop type 1 diabetes. It is an autoimmune disease. Our immune system attacks and destroys Beta cells in the pancreas, where insulin is produced. As a result, pancreas is unable to produce insulin and sugar builds up in our blood. People with type I diabetes are insulin-dependent, which means they need to take artificial insulin to stay alive on a daily basis. About 5-10% of people with diabetes have this type.

Type 2 Diabetes: It is also known as non-insulin dependent diabetes or adult-onset diabetes, since it typically develops after age 35. Type 2 diabetes occurs when our body becomes resistant to **insulin** and hinders the way the body uses insulin. While the pancreas still produce insulin, the cells in our body do not respond to it as efficiently as they once did. This is the most common type of diabetes. About 90-95 % of people with diabetes have this type. The onset of type 2 diabetes is usually slower and the symptoms are often not noticeable. For these reasons, many people ignore the early signs.

Diabetes and Erectile Dysfunction

Type 2 diabetes is reaching pandemic levels and young-onset type 2 diabetes is becoming increasingly more and more common. Erectile dysfunction is a common and distressing complication of diabetes. The pathophysiology of diabetogenic ED is significantly different to nondiabetic ED.

ED is often the first sign of diabetes. In large number of cases of diabetes, it remains under-recognized, under-discussed, and left untreated… although it is one of the most 'treatable' complications of diabetes. It affects both - the patient and his partner.

Men with diabetes tend to develop erectile dysfunction 10 to 15 years earlier than those without diabetes. This makes it mandatory for a treating doctor to first rule out diabetes when the patient comes with the complaint of erectile dysfunction. It is also equally important for a treating diabetologist to ask the known diabetic patient about his erectile ability.

The prevalence of erectile dysfunction in diabetes ranges from 35%-75% for those who are below the age of 70. Above age 70, there is almost 95% possibility of having difficulty with erectile dysfunction in diabetic men.

The incidence of erectile dysfunction is about 30% lower in type 2 diabetes than in type 1. The frequency of erectile dysfunction in diabetics also appears to be related to the duration of diabetes for both type 1 and type 2 diabetics. As men with diabetes age, erectile dysfunction becomes even more common.

Furthermore, the risk of erectile dysfunction is even higher in overweight or obese men with a higher body mass index.

What causes erectile dysfunction in diabetes

The causes of erectile dysfunction in men with diabetes are multifactorial and rather complex, although the relative significance of these factors is not very clear. Human sexual response needs wide range of body functions to work promptly, properly and collectively. Diabetes and even the treatment for diabetes affects many of these body functions, thus affecting sexual response.

To get a satisfactory penile erection, man needs normal levels of male hormones, desire for sex, healthy nerves and healthy blood vessels. Diabetes damages the blood vessels and nerves that control erection. Therefore, even if a person has normal levels of male hormones and the desire to have sex, he still may not be able to achieve a firm erection.

Medical science has identified several possible causes of erectile dysfunction in diabetes.

- **Damage to blood vessels:** Raised level of blood sugar in diabetes damages small blood vessels in the body. This is called as 'microvascular disease'. Damage to small blood vessels in the penis makes it difficult to get and maintain an erection. That is the reason ED is worse in men with uncontrolled long-standing diabetes.

- **Diabetic Neuropathy:** One of the most common complications of diabetes is nerve damage known as neuropathy. 60% to 70% of people with diabetes have some degree of neuropathy. A message or an order to get ready for sex and enjoy the sexual act comes from brain via nerves. Diabetic neuropathy adversely affects neurotransmission, which in turn hampers the execution of the order. While erection is a function of the parasympathetic nervous system; orgasm and ejaculation are controlled by the sympathetic system. Neuropathy affecting either system can cause erectile dysfunction.

- **Nitric oxide inhibition:** Nitric oxide plays a key role in the mechanism of erection. Normally, when a man becomes sexually aroused, nitric oxide is released into his bloodstream. This nitric oxide makes the arteries and the muscles in the penis to relax, which allows more blood to flow into the penis. This gives the man an erection. When blood sugar levels get high, less nitric oxide is produced. Moreover, the presence of glycosylated end-products (chemicals associated with diabetes) has been shown to decrease the activity of nitric oxide in the body and may also affect the response of blood vessels to nitric oxide. This results into not enough blood flowing into the penis to get or keep an erection.

- **Low testosterone levels:** Diabetes hampers production of testosterone. About 25% men with diabetes have low testosterone levels. Low testosterone can lead to erectile dysfunction.

- **Depression:** When diagnosed with diabetes, some me start feeling anxious, worried and even depressed due to the stress of having to live with a chronic disease and manage new lifestyle of diet control, regular physical exercise, daily medications, more disciplined living and some other lifestyle changes. This can lead to him having superadded psychogenic erectile dysfunction. A worried, anxious and depressed man experiences low desire for sex, as his mind is preoccupied with these negative emotions. Any experience of not being able to achieve satisfactory erection further adds to the performance anxiety, lack of confidence, loss of self-esteem and thus low impetus to initiate sex or respond to sexual advances.

- **Medication side effects:** Many men who have diabetes are treated with multiple medications to manage impending complications of diabetes and treat comorbid conditions such as hypertension, hyperlipidemia, obesity, compromised kidney and/or liver functions etc. Some of these medications can also lead to erectile dysfunction.

Kindly note: A rather uncommon condition called **Diabetes Insipidus** is not related to Diabetes Mellitus, while it has a similar name. It is a completely different condition in which our kidneys start removing excessive fluid from our body.

Treatment of Diabetogenic Erectile Dysfunction

The treatment of diabetogenic erectile dysfunction begins with the meticulous assessment, and systematic management of Diabetes, to achieve good and consistent glycemic control (blood sugar level). Regular follow-up on an on-going basis is also a very important aspect of diabetes management.

Once a good glycemic control is achieved and maintained through life-style changes, diet control, regular exercise and anti-diabetic medications, all these measures improve the erection quality in many cases. However, additional measures may certainly be required in a large number of cases on diabetogenic ED.

The additional measures to treat diabetogenic ED are discussed in earlier chapters.

Chapter 13
Priapism

Prolonged Painful Erection

Priapism is a **persistent, usually painful,** prolonged **erection** (full or partial) that occurs without sexual stimulation and lasts for more than four hours. If the condition is not treated immediately, it can lead to scarring and permanent damage to the organ including erectile dysfunction.

Priapism most commonly affects males in their 30s and older, however it can begin in childhood for males with sickle cell disease. It occurs in about 1 in 20,000 to 1 in 100,000 males per year.

Normally, an erection occurs in response to psychological or physical stimulation. This stimulation causes certain smooth muscles to relax, increasing blood flow to spongy penile tissues in the penis, producing erection. Once stimulation is stopped, the blood flows out and the penis returns to its flaccid nonrigid state.

Priapism occurs when some part of this system (the blood, blood vessels, smooth muscles or nerves) alters normal in and out flow of blood, and an erection persists longer.

There are two main types of Priapism:

- **Low-flow or ischemic priapism:** It develops when blood in the penis gets trapped and is unable to drain or there is a problem with the contraction of smooth muscles within the erectile tissue of the penis. It is the more common type of priapism and requires immediate medical care to prevent complications caused by not getting enough oxygen to the penile tissue. In most cases, there is no clear cause, however it may occur in men with sickle-cell disease, leukaemia or even malaria.

- **High-flow or non-ischemic priapism:** This type is quite rare as compared to low-flow priapism. It is also less painful. It occurs when an injury to the penis or the perineum, causes rupture of an artery, which then obstructs blood in the penis from moving normally.

Stuttering Priapism: Also known as intermittent or recurrent priapism. It is a variant of ischemic priapism. It is rather uncommon, however may begin in childhood. It causes repetitive episodes of prolonged erections and includes episodes of ischemic priapism. It occurs in males who have sickle cell disease. Sickle cells are capable of blocking the blood vessels in the penis. In some cases, the condition starts off with unexpected and unwanted erections of short duration and might progress over time to more-frequent and more-prolonged painful erections.

Causes of Priapism

1. **Sickle Cell Anemia:** About 42% of men with sickle cell disease will get priapism at some point. (Sickle cell disease is an inherited disorder characterized by abnormally shaped red blood cells)

2. Hematologic Dyscrasias: Other blood diseases such as thalassemia and multiple myeloma
3. Metabolic disorders including gout or amyloidosis
4. An injury to the spinal cord or the genital area
5. Cancers that affect the penis and prevent blood from flowing out of the area
6. Carbon monoxide poisoning

7. Scorpion stings and Black widow spider bites
8. Using street drugs like cocaine and marijuana

9. **Medications:** Wide range of medications are documented to trigger Priapism. The list is given below:

- Medications injected directly into the penis to treat ED, such as papaverine, alprostadil, phentolamine and others

- Medications used to treat anxiety or psychotic disorders, such as clozapine, chlorpromazine, hydroxyzine, lithium, olanzapine, risperidone and thioridazine

  - Antidepressants, such as bupropion, fluoxetine, sertraline and trazodone.

- Medications used to treat attention-deficit/hyperactivity disorder (ADHD), such as atomoxetine and methylphenidate.

  - Alpha blockers including doxazosin, prazosin, tamsulosin and terazosin.

  - Blood thinners, such as heparin and warfarin

  - Hormones such as testosterone or gonadotropin-releasing hormone.

Signs and symptoms:

- Erection lasting for more than four hours, unrelated to sexual stimulation
- Rigid penile shaft, but the glans penis is soft
- Progressively worsening penile pain

Diagnosis

The diagnosis is often based on the history of the condition and a physical exam.

Colour doppler ultrasound can help to differentiate between low-flow (ischemic) and high-flow (non-ischemic) type of priapism. It is a non-invasive, highly sensitive and widely available modality. In low-flow (ischemic) priapism, the flow in the cavernous arteries is either reduced or absent. As the condition progresses, there is an increase in echogenicity of the corpora cavernosa, due to tissue oedema. Eventually, changes in the echotexture of the corpora cavernosa can be seen due to the fibrotic transformation caused by tissue anoxia. In high-flow (non-ischemic) priapism normal or increased, turbulent blood flow is observed in the cavernous arteries. The area surrounding the fistula shows an irregular hypoechoic lesion in the cavernous tissue.

Blood gas testing of the blood from the Corpora Cavernosa of the penis can help in the diagnosis. If the low flow (**ischemic**) type of priapism is present, the blood typically has a low pH, while if the high flow (non-ischemic) type is present, the pH is invariably normal.

Testing a person to rule out a 'hemoglobinopathy' can also be done.

Treatment options

The goal of any treatment for the condition is to make the erection go away and prevent ED. Options include:

- If you think you have priapism, don't try to treat it yourself. Instead, get emergency care as soon as possible.

- **Ice packs:** It helps to bring down swelling in cases of high-flow priapism.

- **Removing the blood:** Under a local anesthesia, a needle is inserted into the shaft of penis (Corpora Cavernosa) to drain blood from the area to relieve pressure and swelling.

- **Medicines:** For low-flow priapism, alpha-agonists can be injected into the penis. They make the blood vessels narrow, thus reducing the amount of blood coming to the area and easing the swelling.

- **Arterial Embolization:** The blood vessel that is causing the problem is blocked in this procedure. This is used for high-flow priapism.

- **Surgical Ligation:** When a ruptured artery causes priapism, a surgeon may do an operation to tie it off. This is also used for high-flow priapism.

- **Surgical shunt:** In this surgical procedure, a surgeon creates a passageway in the penis to allow the blood to drain. The procedure is used in cases of low-flow priapism. There is a high risk of developing erectile dysfunction after this procedure.

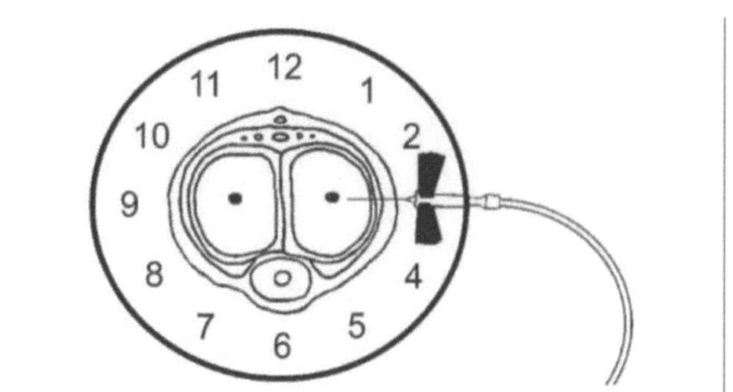

Prognosis

- Most people who develop priapism recover completely when they get quick treatment. Longer you go without medical care, higher is the risk of lasting problems of tissue damage and/or erectile dysfunction.

Priapism in females i.e., prolonged painful erection of the **clitoris** is significantly rarer than in men. It is also known as **clitorism**. It is often associated with persistent genital arousal disorder (PGAD). Very few case reports of women experiencing clitoral priapism exist.

Chapter 14
Aphrodisiacs

Discussing the most popular sexual myth

The biggest and most popular myth that has survived down the ages is about 'aphrodisiacs'. Centuries ago, people believed that aphrodisiacs had magical powers to open up the gates of divine sexual pleasures and fantasies. That belief exists even today. Almost in every corner of the world people still use aphrodisiacs to rev up their sex lives. It could be something as ordinary as banana or vanilla or as absurd as zebra tongue or tiger penis. All kinds of common and peculiar foods, beverages, drugs, magical potions, and chemical concoctions have been tried as aphrodisiacs to enhance sexual pleasure, energy and drive.

Named after 'Aphrodite', the Greek goddess of love, beauty and fertility, 'Aphrodisiacs' are those substances that supposedly induce or boost sexual desire in a person. Several herbs, chemicals, plants, drugs, foodstuffs, and other substances are claimed to have positive effects on the human sexual function. However, there is no scientific evidence to back this up. Also, many so-called aphrodisiacs can be potentially toxic and thus be harmful. It is absolutely not advisable to try anything without scrupulously researching it first, although it may be difficult to find authentic and accurate information because of a lack of scientific evidence on the efficacy and safety of certain substances in human beings.

Non-prescription drugs, vitamins, plants, herbs and supplements that claim to enhance sexual function or alleviate erectile problems are mostly found to be ineffective.

Some of the popular foods that people have consumed as aphrodisiacs are oysters, bananas, asparagus, carrots, avocados, etc. People have traditionally endowed them with aphrodisiacal properties probably because of their resemblance to sexual organs. Garlic is another widely accepted stimulant. So are nutmeg and almond. According to stories, application of almond paste awakens passion in a female, just as the scent and flavour of vanilla is said to increase lust.

Chocolate is universally appreciated as an aphrodisiac. The two chemicals present in chocolate which are being closely studied are serotonin and phenylethylamine. They are believed to create feelings of ecstasy and unbridled bliss.

Plenty of references have been made to aphrodisiacs in ancient literature and history. In 19th century France, bridegrooms were served three courses of asparagus at their prenuptial dinner. The Aztecs referred to the avocado tree as the "testicle tree" and in Spain, Catholic priests forbade its consumption. Cleopatra, known for her beauty and amorous exploits, is believed to have used aphrodisiacs like cardamom, figs, aromatherapy and pearls to enhance her sexual prowess.

Most of the aphrodisiac claims are based predominantly on cultural myths than fact. Their fascination continues to this day, as people still experiment with them to boost their sex lives. Most of the existing evidence is very subjective and anecdotal.

In India, musk has long been held as a stimulating agent. In Ayurveda, *shilajit*, the sap of minerals derived from the asphalt rock formations in the Himalayas is claimed to work like an aphrodisiac. Milk with a hint of saffron is given even today on the wedding night to supposedly set the libido on fire.

There are other more prized and deadly aphrodisiacs. For instance, the rhinoceros horns that bears a phallic symbol, is used in many cultures to perk up sexual performance. Zebra tongue and tiger penis is believed to boost your machismo.

There may be plenty of vibrancy and high spiritedness in the world of aphrodisiacs, but delve a bit deeper and all that you come across is disheartening delusion and deception. Aphrodisiacs don't perform miracles. Actually they don't perform at all because **there is no such thing as an aphrodisiac. There is no food or substance that exists in the world that can be called a sex tonic, sex stimuli, sex drug or aphrodisiac. All such claims are misleading.**

People should not be under the false impression that use of aphrodisiacs can set you on fire sexually or can solve all your bedroom problems.

Although countless research and studies are being done the world over about aphrodisiacs and their effect, nobody has been able to prove successfully that aphrodisiacs stimulate sexual desire in human beings. No scientific confirmations have been made yet about chemicals permeating the hypothalamic region of the brain. It is the hypothalamus, a complex region in the brain that controls sexual desire. Thus, it is wrong to make claims that aphrodisiacs work as stimulants and can increase your libido or solve all your sexual inadequacies.

Irrespective of whether or not aphrodisiacs act on the body, the power of 'suggestion', psychologically, is the key. If one greatly believes that using any particular substance (alleged aphrodisiac or not) will help boost his/her sexual capabilities, then it can help bring about sexual desire and arousal at least in the short-term, but this is more psychogenic and a self-suggestion, and the substance merely works as a placebo. Of course, a well-rested body, adequate time, privacy, a conducive environment, confidence in your contraception, a relaxed state of mind, and an attraction for the partner may do just the same thing. Of course, as we always say, 'Love is the greatest aphrodisiac' that never fails, and that has been proven time and time again. What drugs cannot do… Love can. 'True Love' is the most powerful stimulant and aphrodisiac. If the couple does not feel for each other, they could consume all the world's oysters, tiger penis or Spanish Fly, but it will be in vain.

The second most important aphrodisiac, we tell our patients, is your health. If you are in good health, not suffering from high blood pressure, high cholesterol or other diseases, and you are relaxed, you can lead a healthy sexual life. Then you don't need an artificial agent to get aroused. You cannot isolate sexual health from the rest of your body. If you have a healthy diet and maintain good health, you will automatically have a satisfactory sexual life.

Our patients frequently ask us, *"Doctor, which is the best diet for sex?"* And we often repeat this line that *"what is good for your heart is also good for your penis"*.

You'll be surprised to see the large number of ads for aphrodisiacs appearing in regional vernacular papers—all of them desperately wooing customers with promises of sexual bliss. These ads are published by fraudulent companies making cheap drugs, unscrupulous medical practitioners, quacks and others. After reading them, people come to us for advice on the use of aphrodisiacs. They get shocked when we debunk the aphrodisiac theory and tell them something as simple as 'good health' ensures good sexual life. Eat the right food and lead a healthy lifestyle, and you will be naturally stimulated when required. Sexual desire or drive cannot be induced with the help of an outside agent, it has to come from within.

Is Sildenafil an aphrodisiac ?

Effective drugs like Sildenafil citrate (Viagra) and Tadalafil (Tazzle), are now available in India for the complaint of inability to 'sustain' the erection. These drugs also cannot bring about an 'artificial' erection in a flaccid penis. They only help to "sustain" the existing normal erection longer. These drugs are useless in those who have difficulty in 'getting' an erection. They absolutely **do not enhance libido or induce sexual desire**. They help only those who get an erection 'on their own' but cannot sustain it long enough to perform satisfactory sexual intercourse. It is absolutely not advisable to take these drugs without a proper prescription by a qualified specialist. There are risks involved in taking them; and unless one is guided by a qualified expert, self-medication should strictly be avoided.

Downside of Sildenafil (Viagra)

- Sildenafil is effective in only 70 per cent cases. Moreover, it takes up to an hour for the body to absorb it and show any effect.

- Sildenafil is contraindicated in those cases in which heart-disease medications such as nitrate drugs are being used. **The combination of Sildenafil and nitrates can make your blood pressure suddenly drop to unsafe levels, causing dizziness, fainting, a stroke, or even a heart attack.**

- In rare instances, men taking Sildenafil have reported a sudden decrease or loss of vision.

- Sudden decrease or loss of hearing has also been reported in people taking Sildenafil.

- Some men may experience a flushed face, altered color perception, bluish vision, blurred vision, upset stomach or a headache.

- If one has prostate problems or high blood pressure and is on medication such as alpha blockers, Sildenafil must be avoided.

- Priapism, a painful and prolonged erection that lasts for two to six hours, is a rare but potentially serious side effect of Sildenafil. A prolonged erection can permanently damage the tissues of the penis.

- The safety of Sildenafil has not been studied adequately for men above sixty five years of age.

- It is also not medically advisable to take it twice in one day.

Chapter 15
When to Consult a Sex Therapist

De-stigmatising sex therapy

Whenever we suffer an asthmatic attack or a lung infection we immediately go to a chest physician and promptly get ourselves treated. If our digestive system gets dysfunctional, we do not hesitate to go to a gastroenterologist. For a skin problem dermatologists are consulted promptly. Any chest pain and we rush for an electrocardiogram to a heart specialist. But whenever a man suffers from a sexual problem such as *erectile dysfunction* or *premature ejaculation*, where neither can he enjoy sex himself nor can he satisfy his wife, he either deliberately avoids going to a sex therapist, or then he is totally ignorant about the existence of a specialist who is trained in treating sexual problems.

If a woman suffers pain during intercourse or finds herself unable to reach an orgasm, she at the most, may visit her gynaecologist but would never even think of consulting a 'sex therapist'.

Why is it so?

Why do we hesitate to consult a 'sex therapist'? According to us, it's because of three main causes.

We have been taught to look down upon sex and sexual desire as something dirty, shameful, vulgar and condemnable for generations. A person feels guilty if he has a normal sexual urge. Those who consciously suppress their sexual desire and refrain from sex are respected and glorified in society. A young man feels guilty if he gets sexually aroused looking at a beautiful young woman. He feels like a sinner whenever he masturbates or gets a wet-dream. A woman too, condemns herself if she experiences normal sexual urges. It often happens that the husband either looks down upon his wife for her expression of a sexual urge or even starts suspecting her fidelity if she shows active interest in sexual gratification. This age-old condemnatory attitude towards sex and sexual desire comes in the way of consulting a sex therapist whenever one has a query or difficulty regarding his/her sexual desire, sexual capability or sexual satisfaction.

Another reason why people avoid consulting a sex therapist is that there are a number of 'quacks', who pose as sex specialists through advertisements. Many times, these people are unqualified and untrained. They do not even have a proper medical degree. They display either false degrees or unknown degrees. They deliberately propagate myths such as 'masturbation is harmful' or 'wet-dreams is a disease'. Due to lack of proper sex education in schools, colleges or for that matter anywhere in society, a common man falls prey to such fraudulent advertisements and lands up getting cheated by these quacks. We would like to enlighten readers that 'qualified' medical practitioners are not allowed legally to publish or display any kind of advertisement. This simply proves that ALL those who give advertisements of their so-called sex clinics are frauds and cheats.

Serious lack of qualified sex therapists

Unfortunately, there is a serious lack of qualified sex therapists even in metropolitan cities. As compared to the number of cardiologists, child specialists, orthopaedic surgeons, skin specialists etc. we have less than 1 per cent truly qualified/genuine sex therapists even in Mumbai, the commercial capital of our country. This lack of availability of genuinely practicing sex therapists makes it further difficult for a person to take the step towards getting his/her sexual problem treated correctly and in time.

The third reason why people either hesitate or completely avoid consulting a sex therapist is due to a lack of 'clarity' about when to consult a sex therapist?

Women prefer visiting a gynaecologist whenever they have complaints related to their genital area. It is true that gynaecologists are trained in treating any organic (biological) problem related to the genitals. However, very often sexual problems are emotional, psychological or relational in origin and gynaecologists have no training in tackling such a problem. Women's sexual problems such as 'fear of intercourse', 'inability to relax and actively participate in the sexual act', frigidity, 'not being able to climax (orgasm)', vaginismus etc. are not biological problems. Such problems are either emotional/ psychological in nature or have their roots in the lack of proper pre-marital counselling and sex education for both husband and wife. Even qualified gynaecologists have no inkling or training in handling these problems. Sometimes some aware people consult a clinical psychologist or a counsellor for such problems. Unfortunately, clinical psychologists and counsellors are graduates or post-graduates in psychology from the arts stream, and totally lack the knowledge in medical science. This makes them completely incapable of helping those who require sex therapy.

Very often men tend to go to skin & VD specialists for their sexual problems. Skin & VD specialists are undoubtedly trained in treating skin diseases and sexually transmitted infections, but they are not trained in sexual problems such as erectile dysfunction (impotence) or premature ejaculation. They are utter aliens when it comes to treating cases that require sex counselling and sex therapy.

Therefore, one needs to understand when to consult a qualified/trained sex therapist.

Situations/conditions when one needs to and should consult a sex therapist

1. When s/he finds that s/he has either 'no desire', 'low desire' or 'altered desire' for sex. When we say altered, it means his/her sexual arousal happens with subjects or objects other than a person of the opposite sex of a matching age

2. When the sexual desire and need of married partners is mismatched most of the time

3. When a man either fails to 'attain' or 'sustain' erection in spite of appropriate sexual stimulation i.e. *Erectile Dysfunction*

4. When a man is unable to penetrate and perform intercourse during sexual intimacy with a willing partner

5. When a man ejaculates earlier than his own or his partner's expectations persistently on a regular basis i.e. *Premature ejaculation,* resulting in a lack of sexual satisfaction for the partner

6. When a man takes excessively long time to ejaculate or is unable to ejaculate in spite of a proper sexual intercourse with a willing partner

7. When s/he has disturbing doubts and anxieties related to his/her sexual desire, arousal, capability (potency), stamina, performance or satisfaction

8. Whenever s/he has doubts or anxieties about the anatomy and physiology (functioning) of one's own or the partner's sex organs

9. When s/he has disturbing attitudinal issues regarding one's own or his/her partner's role in a sexual act. For e.g. Who should take the initiative, what is the correct technique and duration of foreplay, what should be the correct frequency of intercourse, when and where intercourse should or should not be performed, who is supposed to be an active partner, should s/he fantasise about somebody else while having sex with the spouse

10. When s/he is obsessively preoccupied with sexual feelings, desires or urges that it is affecting his/her ability to perform essential human duties and responsibilities

11. When s/he has urges to engage in perverted sexual behaviours such as sadomasochism and anal sex

12. When intercourse is either not happening or it is painful in spite of mutual willingness, cooperation and active participation

13. When a woman is unable to achieve orgasm at any time or most of the times during willing sexual encounters with a loving partner in spite of mutual cooperation and active participation

14. Before the marriage for a proper sex education session

15. When a person is confused about his/her sexual orientation and sexual preferences

16. When a person is struggling with feelings of guilt/shame regarding sex.

This covers all possible situations and conditions when one should consult a genuine sex therapist for help.

To conclude, in spite of so many problems faced by so many people regarding their sexuality, it is unfortunate that they either do not acknowledge that they have a problem, or acknowledge but do not accept that they need to seek help to address the issue, or they accept but do not take the action of consulting a sex therapist because of the stigma attached to consulting a sex therapist.

It is important in this day and age when men and women are walking shoulder to shoulder in all the areas of life, and when women are gradually feeling more liberated about their sexuality, that mutual sexual satisfaction and sexual health be given the status that it deserves in a relationship, and this is where the sex therapist comes in.

Chapter 16
Frequently Unanswered Questions

Issues around Penis, Libido, Erection and Sexual Performance

PERFORMANCE ANXIETY

Q: I am 32 and I am getting married next month. I am constantly worried about my ability to sexually satisfy my wife on the first night. What do I do? I want her first impression of me to be fantastic. Please help!

A: You seem to be experiencing "performance anxiety" that many men experience before marriage. This is rather common.

Remember, it is not necessary to have sexual intercourse on the very first night. Sex is not the first and the only thing on a woman's mind. A woman looks forward to first understand and love her husband before she is ready for sexual intercourse. The success of a marriage depends on the love and understanding between partners and not on the first sexual performance.

Let her first impression of you be one of a gentle, caring and friendly person rather than one of an impatient and anxious partner.

Everyone experiences some level of 'performance anxiety' in the first few attempts. However, later on this diminishes. In the correct circumstances and in a relaxed environment, with an equally involved and responsive partner, you will be able to perform sexual intercourse without much difficulty.

PEYRONIE'S DISEASE

Q: I am a practicing doctor. I wish to know, what is Peyronie's disease? What are various treatment options for treating this disease?

A: Peyronie's disease (also known as fibrous cavernositis or plastic induration of the penis) was first described by the French doctor - Francois de la Peyronie in 1743. It is characterized by the formation of a plaque or hardened scar tissue (fibrosis) beneath the skin of the penis that causes pain, curvature, and distortion, usually during an erection.

The treatment choices for patients with Peyronie's disease are very limited. The objective of treatment is mainly to maintain normal sexual function and relieve pain. Invariably, surgery is the only effectual treatment. As Peyronie's disease may simply resolve by itself, doctors often suggest waiting for 1 or 2 years before going for this option.

The non-surgical treatment should be implemented within 6 months after the onset of the symptoms and before the plaque has calcified. Para-aminobenzoate tablets (B-complex substance) and Vitamin E capsules can be taken for a few months under medical supervision. A calcium channel blocker such as verapamil, an enzyme (collagenase) that breaks down connective tissue and steroids such as cortisone can be injected into the plaque or delivered by 'iontophoresis'. Iontophoresis is a painless method of delivering medication to localized tissue using an electrical current.

DOES SIZE MATTER?

Q: I am 27. My fiancé is 31. We are getting married shortly. Recently my fiancé made a confession to me that his penis is small in size. He is worried whether he will be able to satisfy me through intercourse. Is it true that that the satisfaction of a woman depends on the size of the male penis?

A: A large number of men carry the complex of small penile size. The size is invariably thought to be the parameter for one's manliness and one's ability to satisfy his partner. A woman's satisfaction does not depend on the size of the penis. On the contrary, too big a penis can be a problem, as it could hurt the partner. Only the outer 1/3rd of the woman's vagina (approximately 2 inches) is sensitive to sexual stimuli. So, it doesn't matter to a woman how deep one reaches during the intercourse. If an erect penis is even 2 inches, which is usually the case with most men, it is enough to satisfy his woman. It is not the size, but what you do with what you have, that truly counts.

In men too, only the 'Glans-penis' (the front portion) is sensitive to erotic sensations. The shaft behind the glans is incapable of feeling erotic sensations. So the pleasure of the male partner too, does not depend of the entire length of the penis, but depends only on the sensitivity (and not the size) of the glans-penis.

A common mistaken belief that a flaccid penis gains in size on erection, in proportion to its flaccid size, causes this fear. Though all penises are different in their flaccid state, they become much more similar in size, when they get erect. Also, one tends to find one's penis small as it is always seen from above, as against that of others, which is observed from the side or from the front. Different angles from which the penis is viewed also makes the penis 'appear' small or big, as the case may be.

BLUE BALLS

Q: What is "blue balls"? Is it a serious condition? Why does it occur? Does having intercourse treat this problem? I am in a lot of pain.

A: Blue balls are a condition very commonly experienced by many normal men. It is characterized by pain, discomfort and aching of the genitals characteristically after the sexual arousal. Though uncomfortable, it is neither a disease nor is it dangerous or harmful.

A blue ball occurs due to the collection of blood, or vasocongestion in the genitals during sexual arousal. Blue balls occur when sexual arousal is not followed by ejaculation or orgasm because the pooled blood takes longer to leave the genitals when ejaculation does not occur. All of these can cause discomfort and pain for the man, which can only be alleviated by an orgasm / ejaculation. Orgasm and ejaculation relieves the build-up of pressure due to this pooling of blood. Masturbation to the point of ejaculation (orgasm) is therefore the fastest and best remedy to relieve blue balls.

Blue balls is also an excuse that some teenage boys use to persuade their girlfriends into having sexual intercourse, claiming that the only way they can prevent the ache and pain of blue balls is to climax through intercourse. Girls need to know that they are free to decline intercourse as men can easily relieve themselves through masturbation.

<u>**PHIMOSIS AND CIRCUMCISION**</u>

Q: I cannot pull back the foreskin on my penis properly. Will this cause any problem after marriage? What should I do?

A: The head of the penis (glans penis) is the part of the penis that is most sensitive to sexual stimulation and has the most nerve endings (neuro-receptors). A man enjoys sexual stimulation better, if his glans penis is uncovered by the foreskin during the sexual act. Ideally the foreskin needs to get retracted on an erect penis, enough to expose the whole glans-penis. This may either happen on its own on full erection or one may have to do it manually before penetration. Both ways are normal and fine. If the retraction of the foreskin is not possible or painful, then it is a medical condition known as "Phimosis". This condition requires a minor surgery known as "Circumcision". However, this should be decided only after a physical examination by a qualified doctor.

There is always the concern of a person developing paraphimosis (a painful surgical condition) if the foreskin is getting retracted incompletely. I would advise you to get yourself examined by a surgeon.

<u>**NIGHTFALL DILEMMA**</u>

Q: So I gave up the habit of masturbating since last one month. Ever since, I have started suffering from nightfall. Does this suggest a problem in my reproductive system? Please help.

A: At the age of 12-13, the testes in adolescent boys start producing sperms. Boys at this age begin to develop strong sexual attraction and feelings towards girls. Many boys start discharging semen while asleep. This discharge is often (but not always) accompanied by sexual dreams. This is commonly known by several names such as - 'Wet Dreams', 'Nightfall' or 'Nocturnal emission of semen'. This is a natural, normal, common, involuntary and uncontrollable response to sexual tension that gets built up in a man's body due to the rush of sex hormones. Don't worry; feel alarmed or guilty about 'nightfall'. It is not a disease and it happens with all normal men. It is absolutely harmless and has no ill effect on one's body, fitness, manhood or fertility.

If you avoid masturbating, then nightfall is almost inevitable. One of these two things has to happen.

A normal man produces at least 20 thousand sperms every minute and the same number of old sperms die every minute too. With this rate of production (spermatogenesis), the body needs an outlet. Either one can ejaculate (through intercourse or masturbation) or nightfall will occur.

Neither is nightfall a disease nor is masturbation. Both are harmless and natural physiological processes.

PEARLY PENILE PAPULES

Q: I am a 21-year-old single boy. I have developed multiple white pin-head-sized spots on the ridge of my glans penis. Is it due to some STD? I have not had sex with anyone. They don't pain or bleed. However, I am extremely worried about them. Help!

A: If you are freaking out over the small, white, pin-head-sized spots that have appeared on the ridge of your glans penis, you can breathe a sigh of relief as these are completely harmless! They are termed as "pearly penile papules" (PPP), also known as 'Hirsuties Coronae Glandis' or 'Hirsutoid papillomas'.

Pearly penile papules (PPP) are tiny, dome-shaped to filiform skin-colored papules that typically are found on the corona or sulcus of the glans penis. They are usually arranged circumferentially in one or many rows. These are often mistaken for a sexually transmitted disease such as venereal warts, but are in fact entirely innocuous. You cannot contract them or spread them. They also do not itch, weep or bleed - but if they do, make sure you see your doctor.

It is believed that these papules are more common in men who are not circumcised. It usually develops in men who are in their twenties or thirties. However, the mechanisms underlying their development remain unknown. In the absence of a conclusive cause for PPP and due to its harmlessness to one's health, there is no treatment required. Under no circumstances should one attempt to remove them oneself. Even so, if you're still concerned, do not hesitate to get examined by a qualified doctor.

PENILE FRACTURE

Q: When I get a very hard erection, is it possible to fracture or break my erect penis? My friends told me that it happens with some men and that it is very painful. If such a thing happens, what is the treatment?

A: Even though there are no actual bones in a penis, it is possible to fracture or break one's penis. It is termed as 'penile fracture'.

Penile fracture occurs when an erect penis hits or bangs against a less flexible and harder place. This could happen if a sexually aroused man enthusiastically and forcefully thrusts his penis into his partner. It could also happen if he over-runs or misses the expected opening of the vagina and instead hits a harder area such as the pubic bone. If the object is tough enough and the erect penis is smashed with enough intensity, the thick membrane (tunica albuginea) covering the corpora cavernosa of the penis can crack, causing an audible sound, severe bruising and pain. This leads to an immediate loss of erection and the penis can be seen to be classically bent to one side or the other.

Penile fractures are invariably a surgical emergency and should be appraised and treated with urgency. In serious cases, it is likely to injure the urethra, interfering with urination. The treatment for penile fractures consists of a prompt assessment and early surgical intervention to reinstate the torn tunica albuginea and rescue the ability to urinate and the erectile function. Like other bone fractures, the faster the broken part is aligned and set, the lesser the possibility of permanent impairment and deformity.

SEX AFTER SURGERY

Q: After my Hernia operation four months ago, I have lost my interest in sex. My age is 35. Do physical illnesses affect the sex life of a person?

A: When a person is physically ill, he usually loses interest in sex and the ability to perform intercourse. Apart from the damage caused to our bodies due to an illness – it is not uncommon to feel apprehensive, anxious and even depressed about the lack of control over one's body. Besides, we also suffer the loss of the benefits of sexual intimacy. This can induce a 'sense of isolation' in the ill person.

Even after recovery from an illness, many men are often unwilling to go back to their sexual life. "It's too strenuous, too risky," they may think. "I might hurt myself". A wife is mostly aware of her husband's apprehensions and feelings and may share his concerns. This is also likely to lead to a decision to refrain from sex or then to have less sex. A majority of the times, the fear is baseless. This may further lead to performance anxiety and thus psychogenic impotence.

The benefits of a healthy sexual relationship can even accelerate and complement recovery from many physical illnesses. The body is revitalized by sexual activity. Endorphins and Oxytocin that are secreted in the body in larger proportion due to sexual intimacy contribute positively to one's overall well-being.

After recovery from a surgery or a physical illness, when the treating doctor grants the go-ahead, the couple must consider restarting their sex life as at was earlier.

PHIMOSIS IN MID 40S

Q: I am 47 years old and married with two kids. I have a healthy sexual relationship with my wife. We engage in intercourse, once or twice a week. However, in past two occasions, I felt a severe burning sensation on the foreskin of my penis and found it difficult to penetrate. On closer inspection, I found that my foreskin is not moving back easily; but with a little effort and lubrication with oil, I was able to complete the act. I am experiencing this for the first time in 16 years of being married. The experience is rather unpleasant. Moreover, after intercourse, whenever I urinate, there is a tremendous burning sensation with most of the urine spraying over my pants. This is disturbing. Please help.

A: Your foreskin (prepuce) seems to be infected and based on your description; it would seem that you have developed phimosis (an abnormal tightness of the foreskin preventing retraction over the glans penis). This occurrence is strongly suggestive of uncontrolled diabetes. Infection and phimosis at this age could be a result of diabetes that has developed and has not been detected and treated. Very often a person is not aware of his diabetic status (blood sugar levels) as there may not be any other accompanying symptoms. More often than not, symptoms are also missed, ignored or misinterpreted. Kindly get your blood sugar checked immediately at your nearest clinical lab.

Irrespective of diabetes, this could also happen due to infection – bacterial, fungal, viral or parasitic. In that case, it would be advised to consult a Dermatologist for further diagnosis and treatment. An infection must never be guessed without proper examination. The appropriate laboratory tests should help with some clarity. Till the matter is medically investigated, it would be advisable to abstain from penetrative sexual activity with your partner as you may spread the infection to her. This can even trigger paraphimosis.

VASECTOMY

Q: I am 43. I have two children. My wife and I don't want any more unwanted pregnancies. I am planning to go for Vasectomy operation based on the advice of my brother. Can you tell me the advantages and disadvantages of a vasectomy? Will this affect my potency and sexual desires?

A: During a vasectomy (male sterilization surgery), the tube that carries sperms (Vas Deferens) from each testicle is cut, clamped or sealed. This stops sperms from mixing with the semen that is ejaculated from the penis. An ovum (egg) cannot be fertilized when there are no sperms in the semen. Post-surgery, the testicles will still continue to produce sperms for the rest of your life.

However, the sperms are re-absorbed by the body. As the tubes before the seminal vesicles and prostate are blocked, one still continues to ejaculate approximately the same amount of semen. One's sex drive and erection remain absolutely unchanged after this surgery.

Sexual desire and erectile function remains unaffected after this surgery.

Sexual desire originates in the sex centre situated at the base of the brain. The sex centre is activated by the senses of touch, sight, smell and thought. None of these things are affected by the sterilization surgery. Sexual desire is also controlled by hormones, which remain intact after a vasectomy. The hormone 'Testosterone' though secreted in the testes, directly enters into the blood and does not go through the vas deferens. Neither the sexual desire nor the erectile ability (potency) is affected by a vasectomy.

Advantages: Vasectomy is a 'permanent' method of contraception (a birth control method). Once your semen does not contain sperms, you need not worry about using any other contraceptive. It is a shorter, safer and cheaper procedure than the 'tubal ligation' surgery in women. It also causes lesser complications than 'tubal ligation'

Disadvantages: The surgery may cause bleeding or infection under the skin, which may cause redness, swelling or bruising. In extremely rare cases, the vas deferens grows back together (recanalization), and the man becomes fertile again.

CUTS DURING INTERCOURSE

Q: We are married for two years but whenever we have sex, I get small and painful abrasions and cuts on my penis. My wife too complains that her vagina burns after sex. What should we do to prevent this or fix this?

A: A lack of adequate lubrication is invariably the main cause for such complaints. Early penetration while the vagina is still dry can cause these cuts. Engage in relaxed and prolonged foreplay for at least 20 minutes before intercourse, so that lubrication from both sides is adequate.

Good foreplay is the key. This happens when both partners are willing to and enjoy pleasuring each other. Adequate foreplay will produce natural lubrication, and that will solve the problem.

REFRACTORY PERIOD

Q: I am a 29-year-old happily married man. I am very faithful to my wife. We have a fairly active sex life. I wanted to know that how long after one ejaculation can a healthy man get a second good erection. Can the second erection be as good as the first one? We tend to have sex multiple times in one night and this is something that's been on my mind for a while. Can you advise?

A: When a man is having sex, his 'endorphin' levels are very high. Almost immediately after ejaculation, he goes through a 'refractory phase' in which he loses his erection, he crashes and all his systems gear down. He feels tired and drained and needs some time to physically recover. This happens to all men after ejaculation. The refractory phase varies from man to man depending on factors such as his health and age. However, after the refractory period, which could be anything from 20 minutes to a few hours, one can get an equally good erection once again. The level of second erection depends on the level of sexual excitement and stimulation.

SEX AFTER ANGIOPLASTY

Q: I am 61 and underwent angioplasty for two coronary blocks about 4 months back. I avoided sex for these 4 months. I'm keen to know if I can start sexual activity now. If not now, then when? Do I need to take permission from my cardiologist before resuming my sex life?

A: Your cardiologist would be the best person to answer this question. In uncomplicated cases of coronary artery disease, cardiologists invariably allow and even encourage the patient to resume all normal activities immediately after the angioplasty. If your cardiologist has allowed you to walk a mile or if you are able to climb a flight of stairs without distress, then you can safely have sex.

Many cardiologists avoid talking about sex with their patients and couples are reluctant to bring up the subject in front of them or even with each other sometimes.

I once met a cardiologist who expressed his fear to me about imagining one of his young cardiac patients dying of a heart attack during sex. He felt responsible for his patients. He spoke to me at great length about the guilt and it occurred to me that there is still a lot of awkwardness and a great taboo associated with talking freely about sex between many doctors and patients.

Sometimes couples are afraid to talk to each other about their feelings, fears, needs and concerns as well. This is a problem.

Four months have passed since your angioplasty. Angioplasty has opened up your coronary arteries and has made your heart function normally. If you are on regular exercise regime and back to all your usual physical activities - at home and at the work place and if you are feeling comfortable and healthy, there is no reason for you to hold yourself back in sex.

SEX AFTER PROSTATE SURGERY

Q: I am 67. I had my prostate removed 7 months back. Since then, I have found that I do not get an erection at all when I am sexually excited. I really want to have sex with my wife. I was also detected with two partial coronary artery blocks. I feel like my health is getting compromised. Will Viagra or Levitra help me?

A: A prostate removal surgery such as a "radical prostatectomy" can cause injury to the pelvic nerves resulting into neurogenic erectile dysfunction. The incidence of erectile dysfunction after radical prostatectomy depends on whether a "nerve-sparing" surgical procedure was performed or not. Reported rates of erectile dysfunction after bilateral nerve-sparing radical prostatectomy range from 18 to 82%. Other factors related to disease or surgery can also affect erectile function.

You said that you are over 69 and have partial blockage of coronary arteries. In that case, you may be either already on 'nitrate' preparations which are usually given in cases of anginal pain. This is common with partial coronary blocks. This makes it very risky for you to take either Sildenafil (Viagra) or Tadalafil for erectile dysfunction. The combination of Sildenafil and Nitrates can make your blood pressure suddenly drop to unsafe (even fatal) levels causing dizziness, fainting – thus resulting in a heart attack or stroke. I do not wish to scare you but the above factors need to be kept in mind. In addition, the safety of Sildenafil or Tadalafil has not been studied adequately for men above sixty five years of age. You're welcome to go and discuss the matter with your family doctor or with a qualified sexologist for further clarity.

PENILE CONSTRICTING DEVICE

Q: My husband has brought a special rubber ring from Hong Kong that he says has to be worn on the penis. I've never seen something like this before. He wishes to use it to have a better and longer erection during sex. He is not very clear as to how to use it. Is this ring dangerous? He says it is safe. I am concerned!

A: These are called 'penile constricting devices'. It is true, they do work, but at the same time they can be rather dangerous if they are left on for too long.

To use the ring, a man must hook his two index fingers into the ring and expand it as much as possible as he would then proceed to roll it down to the base of his penis and leave it on there. This ring can only be used when a man has a full erection. The ring acts as a constricting device that traps the blood in a man's penis, so that he is able to sustain his erection for much longer. It is advisable not to leave the ring on for more than 20-30 minutes. While the ring is on, there is no circulation of fresh blood to the penis. Fresh blood that rushes into the penis brings with it oxygen and much needed nutrition to the penis. So after the ring has been put on for a while, the tissue in his penis starts to die since no fresh blood can reach it. This is not desirable at all. Getting the ring off can be uncomfortable as well, as the man will now have to hook his fingers under the ring to expand it – so it can come off. Moreover, it this process– the ring may snag and pull pubic hair that could be extremely painful.

THE EFFECTS OF ABSTAINING

Q: If a man in the prime of his youth doesn't have sex with a partner for more than 3 years, does it negatively impact his sexual capability, health or lifespan?

A: Most men and women abstain from partner sex at some point or another in their lives. These periods of abstinence can be short for some and longer for others. There is nothing wrong or harmful with abstaining from partner sex. It does not negatively affect your sexual capability, health or lifespan. As a healthy man, your testicles produce millions of live sperms every day. This happens irrespective of your ejaculation. It may calm your nerves to know that there are no difficulties with arousal, erection, lubrication, ejaculation or orgasm for those who do not have partner sex regularly.

MINOXIDIL FOR ED

Q: I have read that a 'Minoxidil solution' used for a hair problem, can also be applied locally on the penis for erectile dysfunction (ED). Is this true?

A: The use of Minoxidil 2% as a topical solution for erectile dysfunction (ED) is at an experimental stage. Minoxidil is a potent vasodilator that directly acts on arterial smooth muscles by opening potassium channels. Due to this action, it was speculated to enhance erectile function if applied topically. A clinical trial/study was performed at the Division of Urology, University of Toronto, Ontario, Canada a few years ago. In this study, a total of 21 patients suffering from erectile dysfunction received Minoxidil 2% solution with instructions to apply 1 ml of the solution over their glans penis 20 minutes before intercourse. The age of the patients ranged from 29 to 65 years. The causes of the erectile dysfunction were vasculogenic in 7 patients, neurogenic in 8 patients, psychogenic in 4 and other causes were observed in 2 patients. 4 were diabetics and 2 patients also had clinical evidence of venous incompetence.

19 of these 21 patients (90.47%) had no improvement in erectile rigidity, or the ability to achieve or sustain an erection. One patient experienced a burning sensation on the glans penis after applying Minoxidil. This clinical trial results indicated that Minoxidil 2% topical solution is ineffective when applied to the penis in the treatment of erectile dysfunction. It is speculated that probably a higher concentration, a different chemical composition or a different delivery medium may lead to better results but presently, it is absolutely not recommended for the treatment of ED.

SPANISH FLY

Q: I have read about the 'Spanish fly'. They say it brings about sexual urge. Can I use it to boost my sexual interest? If yes, where is it available?

A: The most famous and potent aphrodisiac of all is considered to be the Spanish Fly, a powder made of ground-up beetle. When consumed, the Spanish Fly is supposed to create an inimitable state of euphoria. This beetle is found in some parts of Europe. Spanish Fly makes the blood vessels around a woman's genitals dilate and throb, giving her the false sensation of sexual arousal. If a woman takes it internally, it causes inflammation and irritation of the urinary tract, which could result in permanent damage to her urinary system.

Luckily, it is not available in India. What is available in the name of Spanish fly is a fake remedy.

ANXIETY ABOUT IMPOTENCE

Q: I have stopped making sexual advances towards my partner because I am scared that that I won't be able to have an erection. This has happened before when I was tired from a night flight or when I was stressed at work and was unable to have sex. This growing gap in our intimacy is affecting our relationship adversely. Please help me.

A: Anxiety about impotence (inability in a man to achieve an erection or orgasm) is one of the most commonly discussed sex-related fears that many men have. Internet forums are full of chat threads on the subject with many a hoax remedy or bogus product capitalizing on this common and oft visited fear complex that so many men have. We hear about this issue every day in our clinical practice.

Ironically, the fear of not being able to have an erection – itself - is the greatest cause of impotence. In 90% cases of impotencies, the cause is stemming from the mind (psychogenic). It is only in 10% cases that the cause is biological.

Just as it is not possible to make saliva, tears and digestive juices flow at will, there is similarly no possible way a man can 'will' himself to have an erection. These things happen on their own in response to situations and circumstances. If you're tired or stressed or worn down, it's likely that you'll have a problem getting and maintaining an erection. This is common and normal. If one involves oneself in 'relaxed' foreplay, without 'spectatoring' your penis (waiting for the erection to happen), the erection will happen on its own accord.

Behind the fear of a failure to get an erection is a fundamental anxiety – the fear of being rejected. With women becoming increasingly vocal about their sexual preferences and disappointments, we have also had some cases where relationships have splintered when men have complained that their female partners were particularly nasty with them when they were unable to perform sexually.

Your partner's patient understanding and co-operation plays a very important role in getting over what may very well be psychogenic impotence. Communicate and invest in special moments of intimacy with your partner and don't rush things. Your body will know what to do.

Miscellaneous issues related to ED

Nocturnal Penile Tumescence (NPT) Stamp Test

The Nocturnal Penile Tumescence (NPT) Stamp Test, also commonly known as the 'Postage stamp test' is an old test that used to be used in earlier years to evaluate nocturnal erections in a workup of male erectile dysfunction.

During our sleep in the night, it is common for a normal man to get about three to five erections in a sleep state that often last for 25 to 35 minutes. This may or may not be accompanied by a sexual dream or feelings. This occurrence is extremely common, normal and healthy.

Whenever a patient or a treating doctor is uncertain as to whether the patient is getting nocturnal erections or not, this simple 'postage stamp test' can be done.

As suggested by the, San Francisco Medical Centre (UCSFMC) of the University of California, the Nocturnal Penile Tumescence (NPT) stamp test involves wrapping four to six postage stamps of any size around your penis before you go to sleep. On waking up in the morning, check to see if your stamp ring has torn along any of the perforations. If the perforated connections between the individual stamps are torn upon awakening, this is taken as evidence of nocturnal erection. If there is no nocturnal erection, the stamps will appear attached to each other upon waking up. However, if the nocturnal erections have occurred, the stamps would look torn at their perforated margins.

While the stamp self-test may be able to provide you with some information as to whether or not you are getting nocturnal erections, it can't provide details as to the duration and quality of those erections.

Although this simple self-test is now considered old and outdated, it may give you with some talking points to initiate a conversation, if you have never discussed ED with your doctor. Moreover, there is no risk involved in doing this test in your privacy.

Yohimbe and Yohimbine

'Yohimbe' is the name of an evergreen tree found in parts of central and western Africa. The bark of yohimbe contains a chemical called 'Yohimbine'.

Yohimbine is an indole alkaloid and works as an alpha-2 adrenergic antagonist. It is also known as 'quebrachine'. In some animals yohimbine acts as an aphrodisiac; however, it does not do so in humans. Traditionally it has been prescribed for erectile dysfunction, however its reported clinical benefits have been very very modest.

In folk medicine, 'Yohimbe' is used as an aphrodisiac. No scientific reports of human studies on the effects of 'crude yohimbe bark' on sexual performance can be found in the scientific literature. Any mention or discussion of the use of the yohimbe bark for sexual performance enhancement thus begins and ends with folklore.

Substances that have purported to be extracts from the yohimbe tree have been sold across the world as dietary supplements. They contain extremely variable amounts of yohimbine, with no published scientific evidence supporting their efficacy.

Ironically, there is a fairly substantial scientific literature is available on yohimbine. Some animal studies did show that it acts as an aphrodisiac in certain animals such as rats, dogs and golden hamsters. However, it is far less potent in stimulating sexual behaviour in human beings. The modern consensus appears to be that the pure compound yohimbine helps in treating certain mild types of erectile dysfunction in some men, however does not act as an aphrodisiac

A 2011 review by Andersson KE says ~

"The effects of yohimbine have been investigated in several controlled trials on patients with different forms of ED, but the effect has been very modest. It cannot be excluded that orally given yohimbine may have a beneficial effect in some patients with ED. However, as a consequence of the conflicting results, it is not currently recommended in most guidelines for management of ED."

It has been largely superseded by the PDE5 inhibitors.

Low-Intensity Extracorporeal Shockwave Therapy (LI-ESWT) For ED

Low-intensity extracorporeal shockwave therapy (LI-ESWT) also known as Pulse Electromagnetic Stimulation Therapy (PEMST) is one of the under-trial treatment options for ED. It is viewed favourably as a way of repairing and strengthening blood vessels in the penis and improving blood flow. However, it is currently under investigation regarding its ability to promote neovascularization in different organs.

As per the August 2010 trial published in the European Urology (Volume 58, Issue 2, Pages 243-248), twenty middle-aged men (average age: 56.1 years) with vasculogenic ED were given LI-ESWT. This pilot study showed significant increases in the duration of erection and penile rigidity, and significant improvement in penile endothelial function. In spite of showing encouraging research in the said published study, the Food and Drug

Administration (FDA) has not yet approved LI-ESWT as a treatment for ED.

According to an official statement issued by the 'Sexual Medicine Society of North America' (SMSNA), there is not yet enough 'robust clinical trial data' to support the widespread clinical use of LI-ESWT. It is still a relatively new therapy, and more research needs to be done to determine side effects, complications, and long-term effectiveness. The SMSNA recommends that LI-ESWT should be used under strict research protocols. Some doctors have been offering LI-ESWT for ED, but use outside of a research setting is considered off-label.

FDA approvals for new treatments are always accompanied by guidelines for doctors to follow and side effects to be shared with patients.As with any unapproved treatment, if one chooses to use LI-ESWT for ED, there may be risks that are not adequately explained, and/or one may be spending a lot of money on a treatment that may not live up to its promises.

Bibliography

Research, References and Suggested Further Reading

Aghighi A, Grigoryan VH, Delavar A. Psychological determinants of erectile dysfunction among middle-aged men. Int J Impot Res. 2014;27:63–68

Albersen M, Shindel AW, Mwamukonda KB, Lue TF. The future is today: emerging drugs for the treatment of erectile dysfunction. Expert Opin Emerg Drugs. 2010;15:467–480.

Althof SE, Rosen RC, Perelman MA, Rubio-Aurioles E. Standard operating procedures for taking a sexual history. J Sex Med. 2013;10:26–35.

Althof SE, et al. Why do so many people drop out from auto-injection therapy for impotence? J Sex Marital Ther. 1989;15:121–129.

Aman R. Bhonsle. How relationship issues adversely affect libido, arousal and erection in younger couples. Sex Traps & Sex Scraps. 2021; Adhyaan Books

Aman R. Bhonsle. How Transactional Analysis helps while counselling sexual dysfunctions. Essential TA. 2018; Notion Press.

Andersson KE, Wagner G. Physiology of penile erection. Physiol Rev. 1995;75:191–236.

Arackal BS, Benegal V. Prevalence of sexual dysfunction in male subjects with alcohol dependence. Indian J Psychiatry. 2007;49:109–112.

Ballard SA, et al. Effects of sildenafil on the relaxation of human corpus cavernosum tissue *in vitro* and on the activities of cyclic nucleotide phosphodiesterase isozymes. J Urol. 1998; 159:2164–2171.

Baltaci S, Aydos K, Kosar A, Anafarta K. Treating erectile dysfunction with a vacuum tumescence device: a retrospective analysis of acceptance and satisfaction. Br J Urol. 1995;76:757–760.

Bancroft J, Wu FC. Changes in erectile responsiveness during androgen replacement therapy. Arch Sex Behav. 1983;12:59–66.

Bosshardt RJ, Farwerk R, Sikora R, Sohn M, Jakse G. Objective measurement of the effectiveness, therapeutic success and dynamic mechanisms of the vacuum device. Br J Urol. 1995;75:786–791.

Burnett AL, et al. Future sexual medicine physiological treatment targets. J Sex Med. 2010;7:3269–3304. A good review summarizing future prospects being researched in the treatment of erectile dysfunction.

Buvat J, Maggi M, Guay A, Torres LO. Testosterone deficiency in men: systematic review and standard operating procedures for diagnosis and treatment. J Sex Med. 2013;10:245–284. A detailed review of testosterone deficiency, including current management modalities.

Corbin JD. Mechanisms of action of PDE5 inhibition in erectile dysfunction. Int J Impot Res. 2004;16:S4–S7.

Corona G, et al. Penile doppler ultrasound in patients with erectile dysfunction (ED): role of peak systolic velocity measured in the flaccid state in predicting arteriogenic ED and silent coronary artery disease. J Sex Med. 2008;5:2623–2634.

Corona G, et al. Testosterone supplementation and sexual function: a meta-analysis study. J Sex Med.

2014;11:1577–1592. Meta-analysis that examines the relationship between testosterone therapy and sexual function

Corona G, et al. Age-related changes in general and sexual health in middle-aged and older men: results from the European Male Ageing Study (EMAS) J Sex Med. 2010;7:1362–1380.

Curran M, Keating G. Tadalafil. Drugs. 2003;63:2203–2212. discussion 2213–2214.

Esposito K, et al. Dietary factors in erectile dysfunction. Int J Impot Res. 2006;18:370–374.

Feldman HA, Goldstein I, Hatzichristou DG, Krane RJ, McKinlay JB. Impotence and its medical and psychosocial correlates: results of the Massachusetts Male Aging Study. J Urol. 1994;151:54–61.

Ferrini MG, et al. Fibrosis and loss of smooth muscle in the corpora cavernosa precede corporal veno-occlusive dysfunction (CVOD) induced by experimental cavernosal nerve damage in the rat. J Sex Med. 2009;6:415–428.

Francis ME, Kusek JW, Nyberg LM, Eggers PW. The contribution of common medical conditions and drug exposures to erectile dysfunction in adult males. J Urol. 2007;178:591–596.

Gandaglia G, et al. A systematic review of the association between erectile dysfunction and cardiovascular disease. Eur Urol. 2014; 65:968 – 978.

Ghanem HM, Salonia A, Martin-Morales A. SOP: physical examination and laboratory testing for men with erectile dysfunction. J Sex Med. 2013;10:108–110.

Hackett G, et al. Testosterone replacement therapy with long-acting testosterone undecanoate improves sexual function and quality-of-life parameters versus placebo in a population of men with type 2 diabetes. J Sex Med. 2013;10:1612–1627.

Hakim L, Van der Aa F, Bivalacqua TJ, Hedlund P, Albersen M. Emerging tools for erectile dysfunction: a role for regenerative medicine. Nat Rev Urol. 2012;9:520–536.

Hale VE, Strassberg DS. The role of anxiety on sexual arousal. Arch Sex Behav. 1990;19:569–581.

Heruti R, Shochat T, Tekes-Manova D, Ashkenazi I, Justo D. Prevalence of erectile dysfunction among young adults: results of a large-scale survey. J Sex Med. 2004;1:284–291.

Huang SA, Lie JD. Phosphodiesterase-5 (PDE5) inhibitors in the management of erectile dysfunction. P T. 2013;38:407–419.

Hull EM, et al. Hormone–neurotransmitter interactions in the control of sexual behavior. Behav Brain Res. 1999;105:105–116.

Jiann BP, Su CC, Tsai JY. Is female sexual function related to the male partners' erectile function? J Sex Med. 2013;10:420–429.

Jannini EA, et al. Health-related characteristics and unmet needs of men with erectile dysfunction: a survey in five European countries. J Sex Med. 2014;11:40–50.

Jannini EA, McCabe MP, Salonia A, Montorsi F, Sachs BD. Organic versus psychogenic? The Manichean diagnosis in sexual medicine. J Sex Med. 2010;7:1726–1733.

Isidori AM, et al. Outcomes of androgen replacement therapy in adult male hypogonadism: recommendations from the Italian society of endocrinology. J Endocrinol Invest. 2014;38:103–112.

Isidori AM, et al. A critical analysis of the role of testosterone in erectile function: from pathophysiology to treatment — a systematic review. Eur Urol. 2014;65:99–112.

Kupelian V, Araujo AB, Chiu GR, Rosen RC, McKinlay JB. Relative contributions of modifiable risk factors to erectile dysfunction: results from the Boston Area Community Health (BACH) Survey. Prev Med. 2010;50:19–25.

Levine LA, Dimitriou RJ. Vacuum constriction and external erection devices in erectile dysfunction. Urol Clin North Am. 2001;28:335–341.

Linet OI, Ogrinc FG. Efficacy and safety of intracavernosal alprostadil in men with erectile dysfunction. The Alprostadil Study Group. N Engl J Med. 1996;334:873–877.

Ludwig W, Phillips M. Organic causes of erectile dysfunction in men under 40. Urol Int. 2014;92:1–6.

Lue TF. Erectile dysfunction. N Engl J Med. 2000;342:1802–1813.

Maiorino MI, Bellastella G, Esposito K. Lifestyle modifications and erectile dysfunction: what can be expected? Asian J Androl. 2015;17:5–10.

Minnu Bhonsle, Aman Bhonsle. Psychogenic erectile dysfunction and Rational Emotive Behaviour Therapy, Essential REBT, Heart To Heart Foundation.

Morelli A, et al. Androgens regulate phosphodiesterase type 5 expression and functional activity in corpora cavernosa. Endocrinology. 2004;145:2253–2263.

Nehra A, et al. Mechanisms of venous leakage: a prospective clinicopathological correlation of corporeal function and structure. J Urol. 1996;156:1320–1329.

Papagiannopoulos D, Khare N, Nehra A. Evaluation of young men with organic erectile dysfunction. Asian J Androl. 2015;17:11–16.

Polsky JY, Aronson KJ, Heaton JP, Adams MA. Smoking and other lifestyle factors in relation to erectile dysfunction. BJU Int. 2005;96:1355–1359.

Porst H, et al. SOP conservative (medical and mechanical) treatment of erectile dysfunction. J Sex Med. 2013;10:130–171.

Price DE, et al. The management of impotence in diabetic men by vacuum tumescence therapy. Diabet Med. 1991;8:964–967.

Rajan Bhonsle, Minnu Bhonsle, Aman Bhonsle. Male Sexual Dysfunctions and the treatment options. What the FUQ, 2019, Leadstart Publishing.

Rajan Bhonsle, Minnu Bhonsle. Importance of sex education & counselling in the treatment of erectile dysfunction. The Complete Book of Sex Education, 2014, Jaico Publishing House.

Rajan Bhonsle, Minnu Bhonsle. Aphrodisiac: the most popular sexual myth. The The Ultimate Book of Sex, 2012, Jaico Publishing House.

Saad F, et al. Onset of effects of testosterone treatment and time span until maximum effects are achieved. Eur J Endocrinol. 2011;165:675–685.

Salonia A, et al. Is erectile dysfunction a reliable proxy of general male health status? The case for the International

Index of Erectile Function–Erectile Function domain. J Sex Med. 2012;9:2708–2715.

Sansone A, Romanelli F, Gianfrilli D, Lenzi A. Endocrine evaluation of erectile dysfunction. Endocrine. 2014;46:423–430.

Schouten BW, et al. Incidence rates of erectile dysfunction in the Dutch general population. Effects of definition, clinical relevance and duration of follow-up in the Krimpen study. Int J Impot Res. 2005;17:58–62.

Shabsigh R. Testosterone therapy in erectile dysfunction and hypogonadism. J Sex Med. 2005;2:785–792.

Shabsigh R, Perelman MA, Lockhart DC, Lue TF, Broderick GA. Health issues of men: prevalence and correlates of erectile dysfunction. J Urol. 2005;174:662–667.

Sundaram CP, et al. Long-term follow-up of patients receiving injection therapy for erectile dysfunction. Urology. 1997;49:932–935.

Virag R, Zwang G, Dermange H, Legman M. Vasculogenic impotence: a review of 92 cases with 54 surgical operations. Vasc Surg. 1981;15:9–17.

Virag R, Shoukry K, Floresco J, Nollet F, Greco E. Intracavernous self-injection of vasoactive drugs in the treatment of impotence: 8-year experience with 615 cases. J Urol. 1991;145:287–292. discussion 292–293.

Wei M, et al. Total cholesterol and high-density lipoprotein cholesterol as important predictors of erectile dysfunction. Am J Epidemiol. 1994;140:930–937.

Williams G, et al. Efficacy and safety of transurethral alprostadil therapy in men with erectile dysfunction MUSE Study Group. Br J Urol. 1998;81:889–894.

Yamada T, Hara K, Umematsu H, Suzuki R, Kadowaki T. Erectile dysfunction and cardiovascular events in diabetic men: a meta-analysis of observational studies. PLoS ONE. 2012;7:e4367.

Zermann DH, Kutzenberger J, Sauerwein D, Schubert J, Loeffler U. Penile prosthetic surgery in neurologically impaired patients: long-term follow-up. J Urol. 2006;175:1041–1044.

Zhang XH, Melman A, Disanto ME. Update on corpus cavernosum smooth muscle contractile pathways in erectile function: a role for testosterone? J Sex Med. 2011;8:1865–1879.

About the Author

Dr. (Prof.) Rajan B. Bhonsle, M.D.

Consultant in Sexual Medicine & Counsellor

- **Hon. Professor & Head of the Department of Sexual Medicine at K.E.M.Hospital and Seth G.S.Medical College, Mumbai (India)**
- **Diplomate, American Board of Sexology & The American College of Sexologists**
- **Member, International Society for Sexual Medicine & Asia Pacific Society for Sexual Medicine**

Dr.Rajan Bhonsle is an Hon. Professor and Head of the Department of Sexual Medicine at K.E.M.Hospital and Seth G.S.Medical College, Mumbai (Largest Hospital and Medical College in Southeast Asia). The Department of Sexual Medicine at the KEM Hospital, is the only one of its kind in the country.

Dr. Rajan Bhonsle is the Founder Director of Heart To Heart Counselling Centre and Dean of the Institute of Human Technology. He is a senior Consultant in Sexual Medicine & Counsellor, practicing in Mumbai since 1986.

Dr. Rajan Bhonsle passed his MBBS from Grant Medical College, Mumbai in 1981. He stood FIRST in the MD examination of Bombay University in the year 1985.

He has featured as the TOP SEXOLOGIST in INDIA TODAY and the BEST DOCTOR in OUTLOOK Magazines for the last 5 years in row.

He has authored eight books on 'Sexuality and Sex Education'. His book "The Complete Book of Sex

Education" published by Jaico is a Best Seller worldwide in this category.

His Marathi Best Seller "Samagra Kaamjeevan" is in its Twelfth edition since its first release by the Health and Education Ministers of Maharashtra. Dr. Bhonsle has also edited and contributed to a Q&A book on Sexuality published by NDTV.

Dr.Bhonsle started India's First full-fledged Pre-Marriage Counselling Centre in Mumbai. He has been conducting Training programs for Sex Educators in English, Marathi and Hindi. He is the first and the only one in India to conduct such intensive training programs for the adult community (Teachers, Social workers, Doctors, Parents etc) to train them to become Sex Educators. He has also been leading various AIDS awareness campaigns for the youth in India.

He has been writing very popular Question-Answer columns – 'Ask the Doctor' and 'Expert Speak' for Bombay Times (A Times of India group publication), 'Let's Talk Sex' for DNA, 'Ask the Sexpert' for Mumbai Mirror, "Heart 2 Heart' for the Afternoon, 'Intimacy Issues' for the popular magazine New Woman, 'Teen Talk' for JAM, 'Sex Talk' for Maharashtra Times (the largest read Marathi Daily from Mumbai), a column 'Baat Ban Jaye' for Navbharat Times for several years.

Dr.Bhonsle has appeared as an expert panelist on several popular TV shows on various TV channels such as NDTV, Times Now, CNN IBN7, Aaj Tak, Zee TV, Star TV, IBN Lokmat, Alfa TV, ETV, Mumbai Doordarshan, Me Marathi etc.

Printed by Libri Plureos GmbH in Hamburg, Germany